Manual on

Pre-Birth Perils

Antenatal Emergency Masterclass

68th All India Congress of Obstetrics & Gynaecology

aicog Delhi 2026

Advocate Innovate Challenge Optimise Globalise

Manual on

Pre-Birth Perils

Antenatal Emergency Masterclass

Series Editors

Ashok Kumar
MD PhD
Director–Professor
Department of Obstetrics and Gynecology
Atal Bihari Vajpayee Institute of Medical Sciences
and Dr Ram Manohar Lohia Hospital
New Delhi, India

Madhavi M Gupta
MS
Director–Professor
Department of Obstetrics and Gynecology
Maulana Azad Medical College and Lok Nayak Hospital
New Delhi, India

K Aparna Sharma
MBBS MD
Professor
Department of Obstetrics and Gynecology
All India Institute of Medical Sciences
New Delhi, India

Editors

Poonam Goyal
Poonam Joon
Sujata Mishra

JAYPEE BROTHERS MEDICAL PUBLISHERS
The Health Sciences Publisher
New Delhi | London

Message from Series Editors

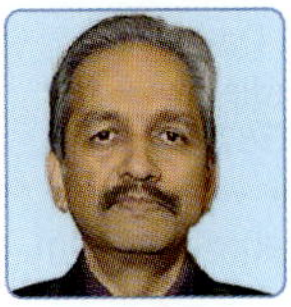

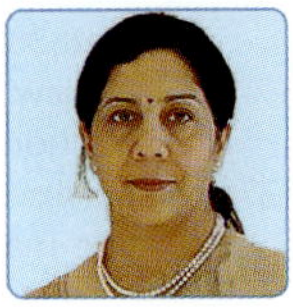

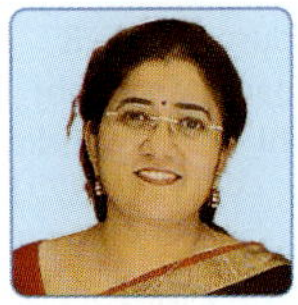

Ashok Kumar
Organizing Chairperson
AICOG-2026
New Delhi

Madhavi M Gupta
Organizing Secretary
AICOG-2026
New Delhi

K Aparna Sharma
Organizing Secretary
AICOG-2026
New Delhi

It is after 18 long years that the 68th AICOG is being held in New Delhi. It is a pleasure to welcome you all.

The Organizing Team have poured their heart and soul into curating an academic program which one will feel a loss if missed. The scientific sessions include both national and international faculty who are stalwarts in their fields. There are 18 workshops with 8 full-day and 5 each in the pre-lunch and post-lunch time.

On this occasion, the workshop faculty, have gone that extra mile to publish the workshop manual for eight workshops. This includes all recent scientific evidence and clinical management guidelines. These manuals will serve as a go-to evidence-based resource in your day-to-day clinical practice. We look forward to receiving your valuable feedback.

We acknowledge the hard work put in by all the editors, co-editors, and the authors, who, in spite of busy schedules and time constraints, have contributed immensely.

We would also like to thank M/s Jaypee Brothers Medical Publishers (P) Ltd, New Delhi, India, for partnering with us.

We sincerely hope that you will enjoy reading these manuals, find this manual useful, and treasure it for future use in your practical work.

We take this opportunity to wish you a memorable time during your stay in New Delhi.

Warm Regards

JAYPEE **Jaypee Brothers Medical Publishers (P) Ltd**

Headquarters
EMCA House, 23/23-B
Ansari Road, Daryaganj
New Delhi 110 002, India
Landline: +91-11-23272143, +91-11-23272703
+91-11-23282021, +91-11-23245672
e-mail: jaypee@jaypeebrothers.com

Corporate Office
4838/24, Ansari Road, Daryaganj
New Delhi 110 002, India
Phone: +91-11-43574357
Fax: +91-11-43574314
e-mail: jaypee@jaypeebrothers.com

Overseas Office
JP Medical Ltd.
83, Victoria Street, London
SW1H 0HW (UK)
Phone: +44-20 3170 8910
e-mail: info@jpmedpub.com

EU GPSR Authorised Representative
Logos Europe, 9 rue Nicolas Poussin
17000, La Rochelle, France
Phone: +33 (0) 6 67 93 73 78
e-mail: contact@logoseurope.eu

Website: www.jaypeebrothers.com
Website: www.jaypeedigital.com

Inquiries for bulk sales may be solicited at: jaypee@jaypeebrothers.com

Manual on Pre-Birth Perils: Antenatal Emergency Masterclass

First Edition: **2026**

ISBN: 978-93-7545-735-0

Printed at: Samrat Offset Pvt. Ltd.

Contributors

Basab Mukherjee
MBBS MD FRCOG FICOG
Director
Ankuran Pluro Fertility and
Fetal Medicine Center
Kolkata, West Bengal, India

Biswajyoti Guha MBBS MD DFFP
Consultant, Obstetrician
and Gynecologist
Department of Obstetrics
and Gynecology
Motherhood Hospitals
Kolkata, West Bengal, India

Devang Bharti
MBBS MD DNB CCEPC GCCHM
Assistant Professor
Department of Anesthesiology
and Intensive Care
Maulana Azad Medical College
and Associated Hospitals
New Delhi, India

Jupirika E Pyrbot
MBBS MD DNB FMAS FICOG
Consultant
Dr H Gordon Roberts Hospital, Shillong
Visiting Consultant
Woodland Hospital
Shillong, Meghalaya, India

Kavita Mandrelle Bhatti
MD FICOG FMAS Fellowship Reproductive
Medicine, Advanced Course in Medical
Education
Professor and Head
Department of Obstetrics and
Gynecology
Christian Medical College and Hospital
Ludhiana, Punjab, India

Mitra Saxena
MBBS MD DNB FICMCH FICOG
Director
Shri Ashwini Saxena Hospital
Rewari, Haryana, India

Neha Kapoor
MBBS MD FICMCH
Consultant
Kapoor Medical Centre, New Delhi
Visiting Consultant
Cloudnine Hospital, New Delhi
Visiting Consultant
Pushpanjali Medical Centre
New Delhi, India

Nidhi Chaturvedi
MBBS MS
Professor and Head
Department of Obstetrics and
Gynecology
National Institute of Medical
Sciences and Research
Jaipur, Rajasthan, India

Pallaavi Goel
Senior Resident
Department of Nephrology
Geetanjali Medical College
and Hospital
Udaipur, Rajasthan, India

Parul Sinha MS
Associate Professor
Department of Obstetrics
and Gynecology
All India Institute of Medical Sciences
Raebareli, Uttar Pradesh, India

Poonam Goyal
MD FICOG FICMCH CIMP
Head
Department of IVF and Infertility
Max Hospital
Vaishali, Uttar Pradesh, India
Head
Department of Obstetrics
and Gynecology
Panchsheel Hospital
New Delhi, India
Chairperson, Safe Motherhood
Committee

Poonam Joon MBBS MD
DMS and Head
Department of Obstetrics
and Gynecology
Sanjay Gandhi Memorial Hospital
Government of NCT of Delhi
New Delhi, India

Preeti Sharma
MS (OBS & Gyne) FIAOG FMAS DIUI (France)
PGDLM CIMP
Consultant (Maternal–Fetal Medicine)
Department of Obstetrics
and Gynecology
Cocoon Hospital
Jaipur, Rajasthan, India

Prerna Keshan
MBBS DGO FICOG FICMCH FIAOG Maters
Cosmetic Gynecology
Department of Obstetrics
and Gynecology
Horizon Maternity and Fertility Clinic
Assam, India

Ranju Singh
Director, Professor and Head
Department of Anesthesia
and Critical Care
Lady Hardinge Medical College
and Associated Hospitals
New Delhi, India

S Arulkumaran MBBS MD
Professor Emeritus
Department of Obstetrics
and Gynecology
St George's University of London
London, UK

Shweta Sardana MBBS MD
Consultant
Department of Obstetrics
and Gynecology
Jeevan Jyoti Clinic and Hospital
New Delhi, Delhi, India

Suyoga Panat MBBS DGO DNB FICOG
Consultant
Department of Obstetrics
and Gynecology
Panat Hospital
Amravati, Maharashtra, India

Swati Singhal DNB FICOG
Senior Consultant Obstetrician and
Gynecologist and Clinical Director
Department of Obstetrics
and Gynecology
Srijjan Super Specialty Hospital
Jamshedpur, Jharkhand, India

Taru Chhaya
MBBS MS FICOG FICMCH FIAOG CIMP LLB
Director
Department of Obstetrics
and Gynecology
Bansal Hospital
Jaipur, Rajasthan, India

Vidyadhar Bangal
MD DNB DGO MICOG
Professor and Head
Department of Obstetrics
and Gynecology
Pravara Institute of Medical Sciences
(Obst and Gyn)
Pravara Medical Trust
Loni, Maharashtra, India
President, Loni Obstetric
and Gynaecological Society

Preface

Every birth is preceded by a delicate continuum where anticipation coexists with uncertainty. The period before birth—often overlooked in its quiet complexity—is in reality, a critical window where vigilance, preparedness, and timely intervention decide outcomes for two lives intertwined. Prebirth Perils dwell in this space: subtle, evolving, and at times unforgiving, yet eminently preventable in capable hands.

This workshop manual has been thoughtfully conceived as a practical and academic companion for clinicians committed to safeguarding maternal and fetal well-being during the vulnerable prebirth phase. It brings together the science of obstetrics with the art of anticipation—recognizing that adverse outcomes are rarely sudden, but rather the culmination of missed signals, delayed decisions, or system gaps.

The manual focuses on real-world challenges: identifying early warning signs, decoding evolving risk, refining clinical judgment, and strengthening team-based responses. Emphasis has been laid on protocol-driven care, evidence-based practices, and contextually relevant solutions that can be applied across diverse healthcare settings—from high-resource tertiary centers to constrained peripheral units.

What sets this initiative apart is its intent to transform knowledge into readiness. Each section is designed not merely to inform, but to empower—encouraging participants to think proactively, act decisively, and reflect responsibly. The workshop format reinforces hands-on learning, discussion, and shared wisdom, acknowledging that excellence in obstetric care is built collectively.

As obstetricians, we do not merely manage complications—we anticipate them, prevent them, and stand accountable for every decision made before the moment of birth. It is our hope that this manual will serve as a catalyst for sharper insight, heightened awareness, and renewed commitment to safer motherhood and better neonatal outcomes.

May this endeavor strengthen clinical confidence, inspire reflective practice, and reaffirm a simple yet profound truth: when we protect the prebirth period, we protect the future.

***Editors:* Poonam Goyal, Poonam Joon, Sujata Mishra**

Contents

1 CHAPTER

Introduction to Antenatal Emergencies

Poonam Goyal

INTRODUCTION

The antenatal period is a crucial continuum in which maternal physiological adaptation intersects with diverse socio-medical variables. While most pregnancies progress uneventfully, a significant proportion may evolve into acute and life-threatening clinical situations that require swift recognition and coordinated management. Antenatal emergencies are conditions arising during pregnancy that threaten the immediate safety of the mother or fetus, often without warning, and demand urgent and decisive action.

India has made substantial progress in maternal health over the last two decades, yet antenatal emergencies still contribute to a major share of preventable maternal morbidity and mortality. The Maternal Mortality Ratio (MMR) remains uneven across states, largely influenced by disparities in health infrastructure, delayed referrals, and wide variations in the quality of antenatal surveillance and emergency obstetric care. In the Indian context, emergencies are often exacerbated by:

- Delayed identification of high-risk pregnancies at the primary care level
- Limited blood banking facilities in peripheral centers
- Coexistence of malnutrition and anemia, increasing vulnerability to shock and sepsis
- High prevalence of infectious diseases such as dengue, malaria, and tuberculosis complicating pregnancy
- Sociocultural barriers and late presentation to tertiary care units

These realities make structured protocols, early warning systems like MEOWS, and strengthening of district-level emergency response capabilities particularly vital. The national focus through LaQshya, Janani Suraksha Yojana, Referral transport systems, and Dakshata has begun to improve readiness and accountability in emergency obstetric care. Yet, continued emphasis on standardized antenatal risk assessment, skilled workforce deployment, and simulation-based emergency training is crucial to reduce preventable clinical deterioration.

Thus, for the senior obstetric practitioner, antenatal emergencies represent not only a clinical challenge but also an opportunity for leadership in improving systems of care—ensuring every pregnancy in India receives timely, appropriate, and safe intervention when complications arise.

FOGSI plays a pivotal role in advancing antenatal emergency preparedness in India by developing pragmatic clinical guidelines, conducting extensive skill-based trainings, and promoting standardized emergency response bundles across all levels of maternity care. Through national simulation workshops in collaboration with ICOG, Jhpiego and government partners, FOGSI empowers obstetric teams in early recognition and timely management of high-risk conditions. Its continuous medical education platforms ensure that practitioners, even in remote settings, remain updated with evidence-based protocols—ultimately reducing preventable maternal and perinatal complications nationwide. Facility readiness is maintained by regular drills.

PATHOPHYSIOLOGICAL BASIS

Physiological adaptations in pregnancy alter cardiovascular, hematologic, respiratory, endocrine, and renal function. While protective for fetal development, these adaptations may mask early symptoms of deterioration. For example:

- *Increased plasma volume and tachycardia* may obscure signs of hypovolemia until late stages.
- *Hypercoagulability* increases risk of thromboembolism, the leading cause of maternal mortality in developed countries.
- *Immunological modulation* predisposes to rapid progression of infections, including pyelonephritis and viral illnesses.

Thus, antenatal emergencies frequently evolve from initially subtle abnormalities that require high clinical vigilance.

CLASSIFICATION OF ANTENATAL EMERGENCIES

1. *Hypertensive emergencies:*
    - Severe pre-eclampsia
    - Eclampsia
    - HELLP syndrome

    These conditions can progress to intracranial hemorrhage, hepatic rupture, or placental abruption.
2. *Hemorrhagic emergencies*:
    - Placenta previa
    - Placental abruption
    - Uterine rupture (though largely intrapartum)

    Antepartum hemorrhage remains a major cause of preventable maternal death.
3. *Thromboembolic and cardiovascular emergencies:*
    - Pulmonary embolism
    - Peripartum cardiomyopathy
    - Arrhythmias associated with structural heart disease

4. *Medical and endocrine metabolic emergencies*:
   - Diabetic ketoacidosis (DKA)
   - Thyroid storm
   - Acute fatty liver of pregnancy (AFLP)
   - Severe anemia with decompensation

   Conditions aggravated by pregnancy often precipitate rapid decline.
5. *Infectious emergencies*:
   - Sepsis (urosepsis, chorioamnionitis)
   - Tropical infections in India such as malaria and dengue can cause shock and DIC.
6. *Obstetric emergencies threatening fetal well-being*:
   - Severe fetal growth restriction (FGR)
   - Preterm premature rupture of membranes (PPROM)
   - Isoimmunization, decreased fetal movements

   Many evolve silently, requiring surveillance tools like Doppler studies and CTG.
7. *Surgical emergencies in pregnancy*:
   - Acute abdomen—appendicitis, pancreatitis, volvulus

   Laparoscopic management is increasingly preferred when feasible.

CLINICAL APPROACH TO ANTENATAL EMERGENCIES

Rapid Primary Assessment

A structured approach adapted for pregnancy:

- Watch vitals.
- Airway protection and oxygenation; maternal hypoxia directly compromises fetal oxygenation.
- Circulatory support with permissive fluid resuscitation avoiding pulmonary edema, particularly in pre-eclampsia.
- Neurological evaluation—particularly relevant in hypertensive crises and eclampsia.
- Exposure to trauma or history of haemorrhage.
- Maintaining normothermia.

Simultaneously:

- Establish IV access (preferably 2 wide-bore cannulas)
- Keep monitoring vitals including urine output
- Perform bedside ultrasound for fetal viability

Fetal Assessment

- CTG for fetal heart rate monitoring
- Biophysical profile or Doppler studies when needed

Maternal stabilization remains priority: *"Resuscitate the mother to save the fetus."*

INVESTIGATIONS

- Point-of-care tests (blood glucose, ABG, bedside coagulation)
- Laboratory evaluation tailored to suspected etiology (e.g., LFTs and LDH in HELLP; D-dimer and imaging for suspected PE)

DEFINITIVE MANAGEMENT

Based on underlying emergency condition:

- Antihypertensives, magnesium sulphate in eclampsia
- Blood products in hemorrhage guided by MTP protocols
- Broad-spectrum antibiotics within 1 hour of suspected sepsis
- Timely decision on delivery when maternal-fetal benefit outweighs risks

PREVENTION AND PREPAREDNESS

Risk Screening

Early booking and structured antenatal screening for:

- Chronic hypertension
- Diabetes
- Multiple pregnancy
- Abnormal placentation
- Severe anemia

Standardized risk scoring tools and referral to higher-level centers improve outcomes.

Protocols and Bundles

National and international guidelines recommend:

- Hypertension and PPH management bundles
- Massive transfusion protocols
- Sepsis bundles

Hospitals must routinely conduct drills and simulation-based training.

Communication and Systems

The "Three Delays Model"—delay in decision, transport, and treatment—remains a barrier. Telemedicine, emergency transport systems, and integration of primary-secondary-tertiary care networks are key strategies in LMICs, including India.

FINAL INSIGHTS

Antenatal emergencies represent high-stakes situations where maternal physiology may deteriorate rapidly and fetal condition can worsen abruptly. Senior obstetric practitioners must combine vigilant risk detection, evidence-based emergency pathways, and timely multidimensional intervention.

Strengthening protocol-driven obstetric care, simulation-supported team readiness, and robust referral systems are pivotal to reducing preventable maternal and perinatal deaths—aligning with global goals for safe motherhood.

SUGGESTED READING

1. Bauer ME, Bateman BT. Maternal sepsis and infection guidelines. Anesth Analg. 2017;124(1):114-23.
2. Gestational Hypertension and Preeclampsia: ACOG Practice Bulletin No. 222. Obstet Gynecol. 2020;135:e237-60.
3. Knight M. Thromboembolism as a leading cause of maternal mortality. BJOG. 2017;124:e1-23.
4. Regitz-Zagrosek V, Roos-Hesselink JW, Bauersachs J, Blomström-Lundqvist C, Cífková R, De Bonis M, et al. 2018 ESC Guidelines for the management of cardiovascular disease in pregnancy. Eur Heart J. 2018;39(34):3165-224.
5. Say L, Chou D, Gemmill A, Tunçalp Ö, Moller AB, Daniels J, et al. Global causes of maternal death: WHO systematic analysis. Lancet Glob Health. 2014;2(6):e323-33.
6. Sinha P. Dengue in pregnancy: Position Statement. J Obstet Gynaecol India. 2020;70(3):169-78.
7. Thaddeus S, Maine D. Too far to walk: maternal mortality in context. Soc Sci Med. 1994;38(8):1091-110.

2 CHAPTER

Eclampsia: The Unforgiving Emergency

Parul Sinha

INTRODUCTION

Eclampsia—the development of new generalized tonic–clonic seizures in a woman with pre-eclampsia—is an obstetric emergency that can rapidly progress to maternal and perinatal catastrophe. Although incidence has declined in high-resource settings, eclampsia remains a leading cause of maternal mortality and severe morbidity in many low- and middle-income countries. Prompt recognition, immediate stabilization, timely administration of magnesium sulfate ($MgSO_4$), controlled blood-pressure reduction, and definitive obstetric management are decisive determinants of outcome.

PATHOPHYSIOLOGY

Eclampsia arises on the background of pre-eclampsia, a multisystem disorder initiated by abnormal placentation and characterized by systemic endothelial dysfunction, vasospasm, coagulopathy and end-organ ischemia. Cerebral manifestations reflect blood–brain barrier disruption, vasogenic oedema, and dysregulated cerebral blood flow that predispose to seizures, intracerebral hemorrhage and cortical irritation. This pathophysiologic cascade explains the need for seizure control, control of severe hypertension, and expedited delivery once the mother is stabilized.

CLINICAL PRESENTATION AND DIFFERENTIAL DIAGNOSIS

Typical presentation is an abrupt generalized tonic–clonic seizure in a woman after 20 weeks of gestation or postpartum, often preceded by headache, visual disturbance, epigastric pain or rapidly rising blood pressure. Any pregnant or recently postpartum woman with a convulsion must be presumed to have eclampsia until proven otherwise. Differential diagnoses include pre-existing epilepsy, intracranial infection (meningitis/encephalitis), cerebral malaria in endemic areas, intracranial hemorrhage or venous thrombosis, metabolic derangements, and tetanus where relevant. Careful history, focused neurologic exam, fever screen and basic labs guide differentiation while management proceeds.

INITIAL RESUSCITATION PRIORITIES

Management is time-critical and follows a modified ABC approach tailored to obstetric care: call for senior help; secure airway and breathing (left lateral decubitus, suction, supplemental oxygen); protect from injury; establish two large-bore IV lines, attach monitors (BP, SpO_2, ECG) and insert a Foley catheter for hourly urine output; draw blood for CBC, renal and liver function tests, coagulation profile and blood grouping—but do not delay therapy awaiting results. Transfer to an HDU/ICU environment is ideal when available.

MAGNESIUM SULFATE: CORNERSTONE THERAPY

$MgSO_4$ is the first-line agent for treatment of eclampsia and for seizure prophylaxis in severe pre-eclampsia. Evidence from randomized trials and guideline consensus demonstrates that $MgSO_4$ reduces the risk of recurrent seizures and maternal mortality compared with other anticonvulsants. Two commonly used regimens are:

1. *Pritchard regimen (IM/IV hybrid)*: 4 g IV loading dose plus 10 g IM (5 g each buttock) followed by 5 g IM every 4 hours.
2. *Zuspan regimen (IV infusion)*: 4 g IV loading dose followed by 1 g/h infusion.

$MgSO_4$ should be continued for 24 hours after the last seizure or 24 hours after delivery, whichever is later. Clinical monitoring of respiratory rate, oxygenation, deep tendon reflexes and hourly urine output replaces routine serum magnesium measurement in most settings. Have calcium gluconate (1 g IV) immediately available as the antidote for magnesium toxicity.

Antihypertensive Management

Severe hypertension (commonly defined as systolic ≥160 mm Hg or diastolic ≥110 mm Hg) should be treated promptly with parenteral agents such as IV labetalol, IV hydralazine or oral immediate-release nifedipine to reduce the risk of intracranial hemorrhage and other end-organ damage. Treatment must be judicious to avoid precipitous drops in blood pressure that could compromise uteroplacental perfusion. Frequent blood pressure monitoring is mandatory after treatment initiation.

OBSTETRIC DECISION-MAKING AND TIMING OF DELIVERY

Delivery is the definitive treatment for pre-eclampsia/eclampsia; however, immediate delivery should be balanced against maternal stabilization and fetal maturity. General principles include: stabilize the mother (control seizures and BP and ensure adequate oxygenation and urine output) before definitive delivery unless there is an immediate obstetric indication; choose mode of delivery based on obstetric indications—cesarean delivery is reserved for the usual indications and not mandated solely for eclampsia; consider corticosteroids for fetal lung maturation if <34 weeks and the maternal condition permits. Active management of the third stage of labor with oxytocin reduces PPH risk; ergometrine and certain prostaglandins should be avoided in severe hypertension.

COMPLICATIONS AND CRITICAL CARE CONSIDERATIONS

Eclampsia can be complicated by pulmonary edema, aspiration pneumonia, intracerebral hemorrhage, disseminated intravascular coagulation, acute kidney injury, HELLP syndrome and abruptio placentae. Management requires multidisciplinary critical care, including ventilatory support, transfusion for hemorrhage or coagulopathy, renal replacement therapy when indicated, and neuroimaging for focal neurological signs. Volume resuscitation should be cautious: women with pre-eclampsia are relatively hypovolemic and tolerate acute blood loss poorly.

RESOURCE-LIMITED SETTINGS AND TRANSFER PROTOCOLS

In settings without definitive care, the consensus is to administer the full $MgSO_4$ loading dose and initiate antihypertensive therapy prior to transfer to a higher-level facility. Safe transfer requires stabilization (airway, ongoing $MgSO_4$, BP control, oxygen and monitoring) and communication with the receiving center. Training, emergency kits, and clear referral pathways significantly reduce adverse outcomes in low-resource environments.

PREVENTION AND ANTENATAL STRATEGIES

Primary prevention in high-risk women includes low-dose aspirin initiated in early pregnancy and, in populations with low calcium intake, calcium supplementation. Early identification of hypertensive disorders through regular antenatal blood pressure monitoring, proteinuria assessment, and risk stratification allows timely referral and prophylactic interventions. Gestosis scoring in the first trimester provides a useful tool for screening and detection of patients who are prone to develop preeclampsia and eclampsia later.

GUIDELINE CONCORDANCE: ACOG AND FOGSI HIGHLIGHTS

The American College of Obstetricians and Gynecologists (ACOG) Practice Bulletin on Gestational Hypertension and Preeclampsia (Practice Bulletin No. 222) consolidates diagnostic criteria, management thresholds, use of $MgSO_4$ for prevention and treatment of eclampsia, and individualized delivery planning. The Federation of Obstetric and Gynaecological Societies of India (FOGSI) Good Clinical Practice Recommendations for Hypertensive Disorders in Pregnancy (GCPR) adapt international guidance to the Indian context, emphasizing facility preparedness, $MgSO_4$ availability, and referral systems. WHO guidance and implementation tools (including Jhpiego resources) complement these recommendations with strategies suited for low-resource contexts.

MEDICOLEGAL AND SYSTEMS CONSIDERATIONS

Given the rapid deterioration that can occur with eclampsia, medicolegal risk is mitigated by adherence to accepted guidelines, documentation of timely interventions, informed consent for obstetric procedures, and clear escalation pathways. Institutional protocols, regular drills, and audit of severe maternal outcomes foster system-level improvement and accountability.

FINAL INSIGHTS

Eclampsia is an unforgiving emergency where minutes matter. Evidence-based, protocolized management centered on magnesium sulfate administration, controlled antihypertensive therapy, maternal stabilization, and appropriately timed delivery saves lives. Ensuring facility readiness, staff training, availability of $MgSO_4$ and calcium gluconate, and robust referral networks are essential to reduce the global burden.

Just to conclude:

- Eclampsia is the onset of generalized seizures in a woman with pre-eclampsia and requires immediate, protocolized action.
- Secure airway, breathing and circulation; apply left lateral positioning, oxygen, suction, and continuous monitoring.
- Administer magnesium sulfate immediately (Pritchard or IV regimens) and continue for 24 hours after the last seizure or delivery; monitor respiratory rate, reflexes and urine output; keep calcium gluconate available.
- Treat severe hypertension promptly with IV labetalol, hydralazine or oral nifedipine, avoiding abrupt BP falls.
- Stabilize the mother before delivery unless there is an obstetric emergency; mode of delivery is dictated by obstetric indications.
- In resource-limited settings give the full $MgSO_4$ loading dose and antihypertensives prior to transfer.
- Prevention includes antenatal risk assessment, low-dose aspirin for high-risk women and facility preparedness.
- Follow ACOG and FOGSI recommendations adapted to local resources to improve outcomes.

SUGGESTED READING

1. Altman D, Carroli G, Duley L, Farrell B, Moodley J, Neilson J, et al.; MAGPIE Collaborative Group. Do women with pre-eclampsia, and their babies, benefit from magnesium sulphate? The Magpie Trial: a randomised placebo-controlled trial. Lancet. 2002;359:1877-90.
2. Federation of Obstetric and Gynaecological Societies of India (FOGSI). Good Clinical Practice Recommendations: Hypertensive Disorders in Pregnancy (GCPR). Mumbai: Federation of Obstetric and Gynaecological Societies of India; 2019.
3. Federation of Obstetric and Gynaecological Societies of India (FOGSI), Indian College of Obstetricians and Gynaecologists (ICOG), Good Clinical Practice Recommendations (GCPR). Hypertensive disorders in pregnancy: Joint guidance document. Mumbai: FOGSI; 2020.
4. Gestational Hypertension and Preeclampsia. ACOG Practice Bulletin No. 222. Obstet Gynecol. 2020;135(6):e237-60.
5. Hull J, Rucklidge MWM. Management of Severe Pre-Eclampsia and Eclampsia. Update Anaesth. 2009;25:50-4.
6. Jhpiego. Prevention and management of pre-eclampsia and eclampsia: Implementation resources. New Delhi: Jhpiego, an affiliate of Johns Hopkins University, in collaboration with the World Health Organization; 2011.
7. Royal College of Obstetricians and Gynaecologists. The management of severe pre-eclampsia/eclampsia. Green-top Guideline No. 10(A). London: RCOG; 2019.
8. World Health Organization. Recommendations on Antiplatelet Agents for Prevention of Preeclampsia. Geneva: World Health Organization; 2021.
9. World Health Organization. WHO Recommendations for Prevention and Treatment of Pre-Eclampsia and Eclampsia. Geneva: World Health Organization; 2011.

3 CHAPTER

Cracking HELLP

Kavita Mandrelle Bhatti

INTRODUCTION

HELLP syndrome was first described in 1982 by Weinstein et al. and the term HELLP refers to an acronym used to describe the clinical condition that leads to hemolysis, elevated liver enzymes and low platelets in pregnant and postpartum patients. It is a life-threatening condition and is considered a variant of preeclampsia. The name HELLP stands for:

- H—hemolysis
- EL—elevated liver enzymes
- LP—low platelet count

It typically occurs in the third trimester but can also appear in the postpartum period.

It is characterized by endothelial dysfunction, platelet aggregation-consumption and hepatocellular necrosis and death. HELLP syndrome is typically seen in patients with severe preeclampsia, although it can occur in the absence of this disease. Preceding hypertension or proteinuria is absent in 15–20% while recurrence in subsequent pregnancies is seen in 19–27%.

Risk factors include age > 35 years, multiparity, and genetic predisposition.

EPIDEMIOLOGY

Prevalence of HELLP syndrome is approximately 0.5–0.9%. Seventy percent of cases occur in the 3rd trimester of pregnancy and 30% occur within 48 hours of delivery. It is associated with preeclampsia in 20% cases. The mortality rate is 0–24% while perinatal death rate is of up to 37%.

ETIOPATHOGENESIS

The etiology remains unclear. It is a systemic inflammatory disorder mediated by a complement cascade. It has similar pathogenesis as in preeclampsia with poor placentation.

There is exaggerated activation of the complement system and hepatic inflammation. Complement dysregulation associated with thrombotic microangiopathy can present as pregnancy-related hemolytic uremic syndrome.

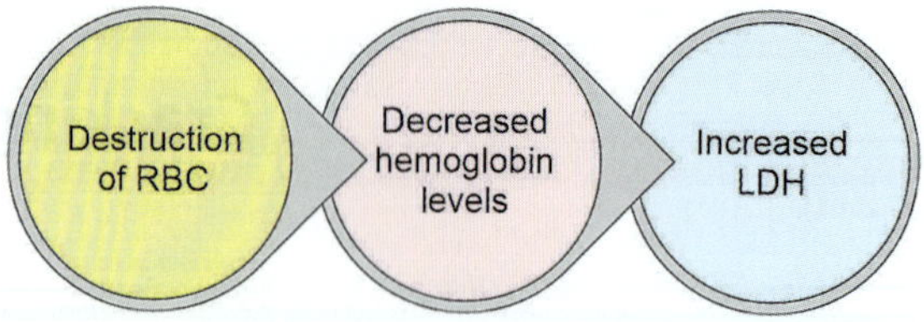

Fig. 1: Hematological changes.

HISTOPATHOLOGY

Hematological Changes (Fig. 1)

Peripheral blood smear shows:
- Spherocytosis
- Schistocytes
- Reticulocytosis
- Anisocytosis
- Triangular cells and burr cells

Microangiopathic hemolytic anemia is diagnosed by presence for schistocytes or helmet cells on a peripheral blood smear. Fatty infiltration, intravascular fibrin deposits, neutrophilic infiltrate, sinusoidal blockage, intrahepatic vascular congestion, hepatic necrosis, and periportal hemorrhage are all visible in hepatic histology. Eventually, this could lead to capsular rupture and intraparenchymal or subcapsular bleeding.

Liver Lesions

There is periportal or focal parenchymal necrosis in which fibrin-like material is deposited. Hepatic changes include fatty infiltration, intrahepatic congestion, intrahepatic and subcapsular hematoma and eventually rupture of Glisson's capsule.

CLINICAL PRESENTATION

Patients with HELLP syndrome may exhibit a variety of clinical presentations. They may present with:
- Nausea and vomiting
- Mid-epigastric and right upper quadrant pain and tenderness
- Jaundice
- Ascites and edema
- Headache
- Hypertension (blood pressure > 140/90 mm Hg)
- Visual disturbances and retinal detachment
- Placental abruption
- Acute renal damage
- Liver hematoma

DIAGNOSTIC CRITERIA

- *Hemolysis:*
  - Abnormal peripheral smear (schistocytes, burr cells)
  - Elevated bilirubin (>1.2 mg/dL)
  - Elevated LDH (>600 IU/L)
  - Low haptoglobin (optional)
- *Elevated liver enzymes*: AST/ALT usually >70 IU/L
- *Low platelets*: Platelet count <100,000/mm^3

Laboratory tests to diagnose HELLP are:

- Complete blood count and peripheral blood smear
- *Liver function tests*: Aspartate aminotransferase (AST), alanine aminotransferase (ALT), bilirubin
- Creatinine
- If liver function tests are elevated—haptoglobin, lactate dehydrogenase (LDH)
- *Coagulation studies*: Fibrinogen, prothrombin (PT), and activated partial thromboplastin time (PTT)

CLASSIFICATION OF HELLP SYNDROME

HELLP syndrome is classified mainly by severity, using laboratory parameters.

Two standard classification systems are used:

1. Mississippi classification (most common) **(Table 1)**: Classifies HELLP into three classes based on platelet count, AST/ALT, and LDH.
2. *Tennessee classification*: More descriptive; requires all three components for complete HELLP.

Complete HELLP

- *Hemolysis:* LDH > 600 IU/L
  - Peripheral smear showing schistocytes
- *Elevated liver enzymes:* AST or ALT > 70 IU/L
- *Low platelets:* < 100,000/mm^3

Partial or Incomplete HELLP

- Presence of only one or two of the above components.

TABLE 1: Classification of HELLP.

Class	*Platelet count (cells/µL)*	*LDH (IU/L)*	*AST or ALT (IU/L)*
1. Severe HELLP	≤50,000	>600	≥70
2. Moderate HELLP	>50,000 to ≤100,000	>600	≥70
3. Mild HELLP	>100,000 to ≤150,000	>600	≥40

- Patients with HELLP syndrome will have normal PT, PTT, and fibrinogen since the condition primarily involves platelet activation without affecting clotting factors.
- Prolonged PT and APTT or decreased fibrinogen can be if there is coexisting disseminated intravascular coagulation (DIC).

DIFFERENTIAL DIAGNOSIS

It is important to distinguish HELLP syndrome from other pregnancy conditions that share similar characteristics.

- *Preeclampsia with DIC:* Patients typically have symptoms similar to HELLP syndrome. Unlike HELLP syndrome, preeclampsia with DIC involves clotting factors and results in elevated PT and PTT. Patients will have proteinuria and hypertension, just like those with HELLP syndrome.
- *Acute fatty liver of pregnancy (AFL):* Like patients with HELLP syndrome, this occurs in the third trimester of pregnancy. The predominant pattern of liver damage in these patients is obstructive. Unlike HELLP syndrome, direct bilirubin is increased in AFLP. These patients have hypoglycemia and increased ammonia levels.
- *Thrombotic thrombocytopenic purpura (TTP):* Fever, altered mental status, acute renal injury/hematuria, hemolytic anemia, and thrombocytopenia are the distinctive features of TTP. There is no impact on clotting factors and hence PT/PTT remain normal. Most patients do not have proteinuria and are normotensive.
- *Pregnancy-related hemolytic-uremic syndrome (HUS)*: They have a TTP-like picture but without fever.
- *Systemic lupus erythematosus flare-up:* Like HELLP syndrome, hypertension and proteinuria may be present in SLE flare up. Hemolytic anemia and thrombocytopenia may be present. Tests for liver function are normal. They have other common lupus symptoms, such as pericardial effusion, pleuritis, arthritis, and malar rash.
- *Antiphospholipid syndrome (APS):* Patients with APS may have thrombocytopenia and hemolysis. Tests for liver function are normal. Like HELLP syndrome, they may develop proteinuria and hypertension. Recurrent arterial or venous thrombosis, repeated spontaneous abortions before 10 weeks of pregnancy, and fetal loss are the main presenting complaints of APS. The diagnosis requires elevated beta-2-glycoprotein, anti-cardiolipin, and lupus anticoagulant antibodies.
- *Fulminant viral hepatitis:* Presents mainly with jaundice and deranged liver function tests.

COMPLICATIONS (TABLE 2)

HELLP is a life-threatening condition with poor maternal and perinatal outcomes.

TABLE 2: Complications of HELLP syndrome.

Maternal complications	*Fetal complications*
Eclampsia	Preterm birth
Placental abruption	Low birth weight
Fulminant liver failure	Intrauterine fetal demise
Acute kidney injury	Neonatal thrombocytopenia, leukopenia, neutropenia
Pulmonary and cerebral oedema	Respiratory distress syndrome
Infection and sepsis	
Disseminated intravascular coagulation	
Cerebral hemorrhage and infarction	
Cesarean section	
Maternal death	

PROGNOSIS

HELLP syndrome is a serious condition with increased maternal morbidity and mortality. Perinatal outcomes are poor. There is a 19–27% risk of developing HELLP syndrome in subsequent pregnancies.

MANAGEMENT

Immediate assessment and hospitalization is required. Women with signs of HELLP syndrome should be managed in a tertiary care hospital. A multidisciplinary management is necessary due to the risk of rapid deterioration. These patients may require ventilator support, vasopressor support, and volume status monitoring. Tertiary care facilities with suitable levels of maternal and neonatal critical care units are the ideal places to manage these patients.

Medical management is mainly supportive, Consultations with intensivists, hepatologists, nephrologists, hematologists and neonatologists should be taken into consideration as soon as possible. Management of DIC, pulmonary edema, acute respiratory failure, and acute kidney injury is necessary in certain cases of HELLP syndrome and should involve a multidisciplinary approach.

Delivery: The only definitive treatment for HELLP syndrome is delivery of the fetus and placenta. This is advised as soon as possible if the patient is 34 weeks or more pregnant, or if symptoms are severe. Vaginal delivery is the preferred mode of delivery. Cesarean section is done in case of maternal and fetal compromise or unfavorable cervix.

Blood pressure management: Blood pressure needs urgent treatment with antihypertensives such as intravenous labetalol, hydralazine and nifedipine.

Magnesium sulfate: Magnesium sulfate is given for severe preeclampsia or eclampsia to prevent seizures and for neuroprotection particularly if the pregnancy is less than 34 weeks of gestation. Continue $MgSO_4$ for 24 hours postpartum.

Corticosteroids: There is no clear evidence of benefit of corticosteroids for treating HELLP syndrome. It is given to promote fetal lung maturation if the fetus is <34 weeks.

Laboratory monitoring: Blood tests are conducted at admission and as per the need thereafter, including a full blood count, liver function tests, and renal function tests. Watch for liver rupture and renal failure.

Blood product transfusion: Transfusion of red cells, platelets, fresh frozen plasma, or fibrinogen may be required as indicated by blood tests and clinical signs. Massive blood transfusions might be necessary. Patients with hemoglobin levels <7 g/dL, should be considered for red cell transfusions. Patients with thrombocytopenia who are actively bleeding should receive platelet transfusions. Fresh frozen plasma and cryoprecipitate is required in patients with DIC. Patients with HELLP syndrome and coexisting TTP will benefit from plasma exchange.

Postpartum care: HELLP syndrome can also occur postpartum and requires treatment and close monitoring. Most parameters improve within 48–72 hours after delivery.

FINAL INSIGHTS

HELLP syndrome is a serious, life-threatening form of preeclampsia with a typical laboratory triad. Microangiopathic hemolytic anemia is the hallmark of HELLP syndrome, and laboratory results are helpful in verifying this diagnosis. Although HELLP is thought to occur on the spectrum of hypertensive diseases of pregnancy but up to 15% of cases do not exhibit proteinuria or hypertension. HELLP syndrome is treated similar to preeclampsia with severe features, but because these patients may be critically ill, they frequently need additional supportive care, blood product transfusions, and admission to an intensive care unit. In the postpartum period, HELLP usually resolves within 24–48 hours. If the patient does not improve, alternative diagnoses must be taken into consideration.

SUGGESTED READING

1. Fitzpatrick KE, Hinshaw K, Kurinczuk JJ, Knight M. Risk factors, management, and outcomes of hemolysis, elevated liver enzymes, and low platelets syndrome and elevated liver enzymes, low platelets syndrome. Obstet Gynecol. 2014;123(3):618-27.

2. Jiang R, Wang T, Li B, He J. Clinical characteristics and pregnancy outcomes of atypical hemolysis, elevated liver enzymes, and low platelets syndrome: A case series. Medicine (Baltimore). 2020;99(18):e19798.
3. Khalid F, Mahendraker N, Tonismae T. HELLP Syndrome. Treasure Island (FL): StatPearls Publishing; 2025.
4. Rao D, Chaudhari NK, Moore RM, Jim B. HELLP syndrome: a diagnostic conundrum with severe complications. BMJ Case Rep. 2016;2016:bcr2016216802.
5. Wallace K, Harris S, Addison A, Bean C. HELLP Syndrome: Pathophysiology and Current Therapies. Curr Pharm Biotechnol. 2018;19(10):816-26.

4 CHAPTER

Placental Abruption

Vidyadhar Bangal

INTRODUCTION

Placental abruption, or *abruptio placentae*, is defined as the premature separation of the normally situated placenta from the uterine wall before delivery. It is a major cause of maternal morbidity and perinatal mortality worldwide, with incidence ranging between 0.4 and 1% of pregnancies. The condition is characterized by sudden onset, often without warning, making it a "silent spike" in obstetric practice.

PATHOPHYSIOLOGY OF ABRUPTIO PLACENTA

- *Initial event-vascular injury:*
  - The underlying trigger is rupture of maternal vessels in the decidua basalis (the maternal side of the placenta).
  - This rupture allows blood to accumulate between the placenta and uterine wall.
- *Formation of hematoma:*
  - Retroplacental hematoma develops as blood collects **(Fig. 1)**.
  - The hematoma expands, causing mechanical separation of the placenta from the uterus.
- *Placental separation:*
  - As separation increases, maternal blood supply to the intervillous space is disrupted.

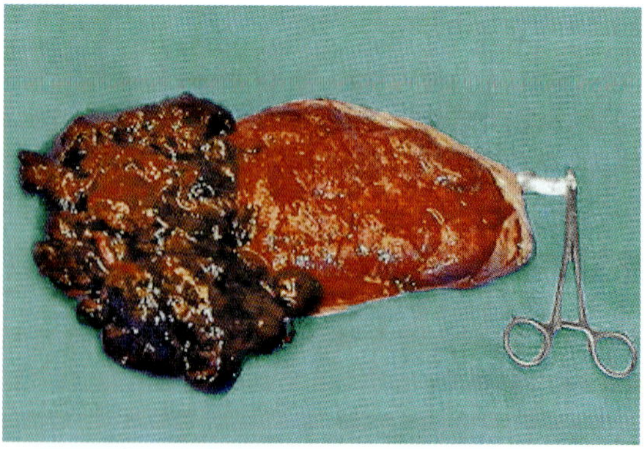

Fig. 1: Retroplacental blood clot in case of abruptio placenta.

  - This leads to reduced oxygen and nutrient delivery to the fetus, resulting in fetal hypoxia and distress.
- *Uterine response:*
  - The uterus becomes irritable and hypertonic due to blood infiltration into the myometrium.
  - This explains the painful contractions and uterine tenderness seen clinically.
- *Coagulopathy:*
  - The release of thromboplastin from damaged placental tissue can trigger disseminated intravascular coagulation (DIC).
  - This worsens maternal bleeding and increases risk of shock.

RISK FACTORS

- Hypertension and preeclampsia
- Trauma (e.g., motor vehicle accidents, falls)
- Smoking and substance abuse (especially cocaine)
- Advanced maternal age
- Previous cesarean delivery or history of abruption
- Multiple gestation and polyhydramnios

CLINICAL PRESENTATION

Typical features include:

- Vaginal bleeding (though may be absent in concealed cases)
- Sudden severe abdominal pain
- Uterine tenderness and hypertonicity
- Fetal distress or demise due to hypoxia

Diagnosis is primarily clinical, supported by ultrasound and laboratory evaluation for coagulopathy.

KEY DIFFERENTIAL DIAGNOSES (TABLE 1)

- *Placenta previa:*
  - Placenta lies in the lower uterine segment, covering or near the cervical os.
  - Bleeding is typically painless, unlike the painful bleeding of abruption.
- *Vasa previa:*
  - Fetal vessels traverse the membranes over the cervical os.
  - Bleeding occurs at membrane rupture and is of *fetal origin*, often catastrophic.
- *Subchorionic hemorrhage:*
  - Bleeding between the chorionic membranes and uterine wall.
  - May mimic abruption but often less severe.

TABLE 1: Differential diagnosis of antepartum hemorrhage.

Feature	*Abruptio placenta*	*Placenta previa*	*Vasa previa*
Onset of bleeding	Sudden, often after trauma or hypertension	Sudden, often without warning	At rupture of membranes
Pain	Painful abdominal pain, uterine tenderness	Painless bleeding	Usually painless, but fetal distress occurs
Bleeding type	Maternal blood	Maternal blood	Fetal blood (from vessels)
Uterine tone	Increased, rigid, tender	Normal, soft	Normal
Fetal heart rate	Distress, bradycardia, or death	Usually normal until severe maternal bleeding	Sudden severe bradycardia, high fetal mortality
Risk factors	Hypertension, trauma, smoking, multiparity	Prior cesarean, multiple pregnancies, abnormal placental implantation	Velamentous cord insertion, multiple gestation
Diagnosis	Clinical + ultrasound (retroplacental clot)	Ultrasound (placenta over os)	Ultrasound with color Doppler
Management	Stabilize mother, expedite delivery if severe	Cesarean if placenta covers os	Emergency cesarean delivery

- *Preterm labor with bloody show:* Cervical dilation and effacement can cause small amounts of blood-stained mucus.
- *Uterine rupture:*
  - Presents with abdominal pain, abnormal fetal heart rate, and maternal instability.
  - More common in women with prior cesarean section.
- *Abdominal trauma*: Direct trauma (e.g., motor vehicle accident, fall) can cause bleeding and mimic abruption.
- *Ovarian pathology*: Ovarian cyst rupture or torsion may present with acute abdominal pain and mimic abruption

MATERNAL AND PERINATAL OUTCOMES

- *Maternal risks:* Hemorrhagic shock, disseminated intravascular coagulation (DIC), renal failure.
- *Fetal risks:* Intrauterine growth restriction, preterm birth, stillbirth.
- Perinatal mortality rates as high as 12–15% in severe case

MANAGEMENT OF ABRUPTIO PLACENTA

Initial Stabilization

- *Hospitalization and emergency care:* Admit immediately to a facility with obstetric and neonatal support.
- *Maternal resuscitation:*
  - Establish IV access with large-bore cannula.
  - Begin fluid resuscitation (crystalloids, blood products if needed).
  - Correct hypovolemia and shock.
- *Monitor vital signs:* BP, pulse, urine output (catheterization).
- *Laboratory tests:* CBC, coagulation profile, blood type and crossmatch.
- *Oxygen therapy:* To optimize maternal and fetal oxygenation.

Fetal and Maternal Monitoring

- Continuous fetal heart rate monitoring.
- *Maternal monitoring* for signs of disseminated intravascular coagulation (DIC), renal failure, or hypovolemic shock.

Delivery Decisions

- *If fetus is alive and in distress → Emergency cesarean section* is indicated.
- *If fetus is dead and mother is stable →* Vaginal delivery is preferred (induction or augmentation of labor).
- *If abruption is mild and pregnancy is preterm →* Conservative management may be considered with close monitoring, but most cases require delivery once maternal or fetal compromise occurs.

Supportive Care

- *Blood transfusion:* Packed red cells, fresh frozen plasma, platelets if coagulopathy develop.
- *Correct DIC:* Treat underlying cause, replace clotting factors.
- *Pain management* and psychological support.
- *Postpartum care:* Monitor for postpartum hemorrhage, renal failure, and infection.

Definitive Management

- *Delivery is the only definitive treatment* for abruptio placenta.
- The route depends on maternal condition, fetal status, and stage of labor.
- Cesarean is common in severe cases; vaginal delivery may be safe if conditions allow.

Preventive Measures

- Rigorous *antenatal screening* for hypertensive disorders.
- *Lifestyle interventions*: Smoking cessation, avoidance of illicit drugs.
- *Close monitoring* in women with prior abruption or cesarean birth.

FINAL INSIGHTS

- Placental abruption remains a deadly obstetric emergency. Its silent onset underscores the need for heightened vigilance, rapid diagnosis, and prompt intervention. Strengthening antenatal care, improving risk factor awareness, and ensuring timely access to emergency obstetric services are crucial to reducing maternal and perinatal mortality.
- Placental abruption exemplifies the unpredictability of obstetric emergencies. Its "silent spikes"—sudden onset without warning—highlight the need for heightened clinical suspicion, especially in high-risk pregnancies. Strengthening antenatal care, coupled with rapid emergency response systems, are critical to reducing maternal and perinatal mortality.
- *Take home message:* Placental abruption, or *abruptio placentae*, is a critical obstetric emergency defined as premature separation of the normally situated placenta from the uterine wall before delivery. Although relatively uncommon, with an incidence of 0.4–1% of pregnancies, it remains a leading cause of maternal morbidity and perinatal mortality worldwide. The condition is often presented in third trimester with sudden onset of vaginal bleeding, abdominal pain, uterine hypertonicity, and fetal distress, though concealed cases may lack external bleeding. Risk factors include hypertensive disorders, trauma, smoking, cocaine use, advanced maternal age, and prior abruption. Pathophysiology involves rupture of maternal vessels in the decidua basalis, leading to hemorrhage and progressive placental detachment. Management requires rapid maternal stabilization, continuous monitoring, and timely delivery decisions based on fetal viability and maternal condition. Preventive strategies focus on antenatal screening, lifestyle modification, and close surveillance of high-risk pregnancies. Early recognition and prompt intervention are essential to reduce adverse maternal and perinatal outcomes.
- *Keywords:* Placental abruption, pregnancy complication, maternal morbidity, perinatal mortality, obstetric emergency

SUGGESTED READING

1. Ananth CV, Lavery JA, Vintzileos AM, Skupski DW, Varner M, Saade G, et al. Severe placental abruption: clinical definition and associations with maternal complications. Am J Obstet Gynecol. 2016;214:272. e1-9.
2. Ananth CV, Savitz DA, Bowes WA Jr, Luther ER. Influence of hypertensive disorders and cigarette smoking on placental abruption and uterine bleeding during pregnancy. Br J Obstet Gynaecol. 1997;104(5):572-8.
3. Ananth CV, Smulian JC, Vintzileos AM. Incidence of placental abruption in relation to cigarette smoking and hypertensive disorders during pregnancy: a meta-analysis of observational studies. Obstet Gynecol. 1999;93(4):622-8.
4. Ananth CV, VanderWeele TJ. Placental abruption and perinatal mortality with preterm delivery as a mediator: disentangling direct and indirect effects. Am J Epidemiol. 2011;174:99-108.

5. Brandt JS, Ananth CV. Placental abruption at near-term and term gestations: pathophysiology, epidemiology, diagnosis, and management. Am J Obstet Gynecol. 2023;228(5S):S131.
6. Cheng HT, Wang YC, Lo HC, Su LT, Lin CH, Sung FC, et al. Trauma during pregnancy: a population-based analysis of maternal outcome. World J Surg. 2012;36:2767-75.
7. Clark SL. Placentae previa and abruptio placentae. Creasy RK, Resnik R (Eds). Maternal Fetal Medicine, 5th edition. Philadelphia: WB Saunders; 2004.
8. Erez O, Mastrolia SA, Thachil J. Disseminated intravascular coagulation in pregnancy: insights in pathophysiology, diagnosis and management. Am J Obstet Gynecol. 2015;213:452-63.
9. Hackney DN, Kuo K, Petersen RJ, Lappen JR. Determinants of the competing outcomes of intrauterine infection, abruption, or spontaneous preterm birth after preterm premature rupture of membranes. J Matern Fetal Neonatal Med. 2016;29(2):258-63.
10. Kramer MS, Usher RH, Pollack R, Boyd M, Usher S. Etiologic determinants of abruptio placentae. Obstet Gynecol. 1997;89:221-6.
11. Kramer MS, Usher RH, Pollack R. Etiologic determinants of abruptio placentae. Obstet Gynecol. 1997;89(2):221-6.
12. Mackenzie AP, Schatz F, Krikun G, Funai EF, Kadner S, Lockwood CJ. Mechanisms of abruption-induced premature rupture of the fetal membranes: thrombin enhanced decidual matrix metalloproteinase-3 (stromelysin-1) expression. Am J Obstet Gynecol. 2004;191:1996-2001.
13. Oyelese Y, Ananth CV. Placental abruption. Obstet Gynecol. 2006;108:1005-16.
14. Page N, Roloff K, Modi AP, Dong F, Neeki MM. Management of Placental Abruption Following Blunt Abdominal Trauma. Cureus. 2020;12(9):e10337.
15. Rasmussen S, Irgens LM, Bergsjo P, Dalaker K. Perinatal mortality and case fatality after placental abruption in Norway 1967-1991. Acta Obstet Gynecol Scand. 1996;75:229-34.
16. Raymond EG, Mills JL. Placental abruption. Maternal risk factors and associated fetal conditions. Acta Obstet Gynecol Scand. 1993;72:633-9.
17. Tikkanen M, Luukkaala T, Gissler M, Ritvanen A, Ylikorkala O, Paavonen J, et al. Decreasing perinatal mortality in placental abruption. Acta Obstet Gynecol Scand. 2013;92:298-305.
18. Tikkanen M, Nuutila M, Hiilesmaa V, Paavonen J, Ylikorkala O. Clinical presentation and risk factors of placental abruption. Acta Obstet Gynecol Scand. 2006;85:700-5.
19. Tikkanen M. Etiology, clinical manifestations, and prediction of placental abruption. Acta Obstet Gynecol Scand. 2010;89:732-40.
20. Tuuli MG, Norman SM, Odibo AO, Macones GA, Cahill AG. Perinatal outcomes in women with subchorionic hematoma: a systematic review and meta-analysis. Obstet Gynecol. 2011;117(5):1205-12.
21. Usui R, Matsubara S, Ohkuchi A, Kuwata T, Watanabe T, Izumi A, et al. Fetal heart rate pattern reflecting the severity of placental abruption. Arch Gynecol Obstet. 2008;277:249-53.
22. Zhang Y, Zuo X, Yuan T, Teng Y. Electronic fetal monitoring characteristics of a patient with sudden onset of placental abruption and intra uterine fetal demise: a case report. Medicine (Baltimore) 2019;98:e15472.

5 CHAPTER

Acute Fatty Liver of Pregnancy

Prerna Keshan

INTRODUCTION

Acute fatty liver of pregnancy (AFLP) is one of the most serious antenatal events documented. It is characterized by commencing from hepatic fatty infiltration to an array of hepatocellular dysfunction eventually leading to dreaded hepatic succumb. Maternal and perinatal morbidity and mortality is significantly high in AFLP as it tends to particularly affect the late third trimester of the gestation. Prompt diagnosis, responsiveness to the altered investigation reports and early intervention is the key toward improved fetomaternal outcomes. If left unattended AFLP may progress to coagulopathy, hypoglycemia, encephalopathy, and hepatorenal failure.

EPIDEMIOLOGY AND PREDISPOSING CONDITIONS

The incidence is as high as 1 in 7,000 to an estimated 1 in 20,000 to be mothers. Carrying a male fetus in the womb predisposes the mother more for AFLP for reasons hitherto unknown. Multifetal gestation and a strong family history of AFLP point toward a genetic basis of its occurrence. However, few of the following predisposing factors can be enumerated:

- Gene responsible-frequent mutations in the *LCHAD* gene, long chain 3 hydroxyacyl-CoA dehydrogenase is implicated in mothers with AFLP.
- Multifetal gestations-attributed to the enhance metabolic requirements of the twin/triplet pregnancies
- Primigravida
- Superimposed GDM and morbid obesity

PATHOPHYSIOLOGY

Although not thoroughly understood yet, it has been hypothetically assumed that the fatty acid oxidation in the mitochondria is defective leading to the deposition of the unhealthy lipids in the liver cells leading to the array of functional collapse encompassing hepatic injury to raised hepatic enzymes and increased serum bilirubin and thereby further cellular injury.

DIAGNOSIS BASED ON KEY FEATURES CLINICALLY

Clinical features can be abrupt in onset not identified till around the 28th week of gestation. Onset of AFLP is mostly beyond 35 weeks and rarely before 30 weeks of gestation. The presenting complaints may be varied ranging from:

- *Nausea and vomiting:* This poses a challenge in differentiating between normal NVP and exaggerated features of AFLP. To diagnose AFLP timely one needs to be AFLP minded! Any nausea and vomiting occurring in the late third trimester should raise an eyebrow of suspicion toward AFLP and needs further workup.
- *Pain abdomen:* Pain in the right upper quadrant is one of the most consistent clinical symptoms of AFLP ranging from mild, moderate to severe depending on the hepatic capsular distension
- *Icterus:* One of the most significant features of AFLP over a quick clinical acumen.
- *Features of hypoglycemia:* Inadequate cellular gluconeogenesis resulting in one of the most initial features of low blood sugar levels, also proves to be a prognostic indicator.
- Generalized fatigability
- Features suggestive of coagulopathy
- Altered orientation and consciousness suggestive of hepatic encephalopathy

INVESTIGATION AND EVALUATION

Although a thorough clinical history and examination is the mainstay of diagnosis of AFLP, certain laboratory and radiological investigation can aid to the conclusive diagnosis. They include:

- Altered LFT—elevated liver enzymes and hyperbilirubinemia, serum bilirubin ranging from 3 to10 mg/dL, elevated transaminase (<500 IU), elevated alkaline phosphatase
- Altered coagulation profile—elevated PT, decreased antithrombin III, decreased platelet, decreased fibrinogen
- Low serum glucose and raised WBC
- Elevated ammonia, raised creatinine and proteinuria
- Ultrasonography—abdomen revealing hepatomegaly

CHALLENGES IN DIAGNOSIS

- It is of paramount importance that AFLP is differentiated from the other two dreaded pregnancy complications-HELLP syndrome, acute viral hepatitis, IHCP, HUS and TTP.
- The key features of segregating HELLP syndrome from AFLP are low platelet counts and hemolytic features.
- Acute viral hepatitis has significantly raised liver enzymes with a different natural history of onset and progression of disease.
- IHCP typically presents pruritus with elevated serum bile acids.

TREATMENT

- Management of AFLP per se is urgent safe confinement not further compromising maternal and fetal health once diagnosis is confirmed.
- Timing of delivery is not dependent on the gestational period considering the dread jeopardy it causes to both mother and the fetus. A multidisciplinary approach with an expert neonatologist and a gastroenterologist, critical care specialist and a nephrologist should be planned to avoid perinatal morbidity and mortality.
- Maintenance of blood sugar levels >60 mg/dL under close surveillance.
- Mother should immediately be shifted to high dependency unit care to provide support related to routine vital monitoring to advanced coagulopathy management and interventional intensive care for anticipated multi organ failure if any.

PROGNOSTIC FACTORS

The most important key to saving lives of mothers with AFLP is prompt diagnosis and early intervention. A delay in management may prove fatal for both mother and the baby. Favorable prognosis can be expected with relevant multidisciplinary team approach and strict vigilance. Relapse and recurrences are rare unless genetically predisposed. Mortality with delayed diagnosis and management can be as high as 30%.

FINAL INSIGHTS

The mainstay of dealing with cases of AFLP is a good clinical acumen wherein recognition of the warning signs are mandatory aided with laboratory investigations. However once confirmed it is the responsibility of the care provider to refer the mother to a center with tertiary level care if not available at the point of diagnosis. Furthermore a team based approach including an experienced obstetrician, expert neonatologist and HDU set up is mandatory for optimum maternal fetal outcome.

SUGGESTED READING

1. Ibdah JA. AFLP: an update on pathogenesis and clinical implications. World J Gastroenterol. 2006:12(46):7397-404.
2. Natarajan SK, Eapen CE, Pullimood A, Balasubtamanian KA. Role of 3 hydroxy fatty acid induced hepatic lipotoxicity in AFLP. J Hepatol. 2018:69(3):709-16.
3. Peng Q, Zhu T, Huang J, Liu Y, Zhang W, et al. Factors and a model to predict three-month mortality in patients with acute fatty liver of pregnancy from two medical centers. BMC Pregnancy Childbirth. 2024;24:27.
4. Rathore RR. International Journal of Reproduction, Contraception, Obstetrics and Gynecology. 2019;8(9):3787-90. Published by Medip Academy, India.
5. Zarni S, Viegas A. AFLP: Literature review. Cureus. 2025:17(10):e94576.

6 CHAPTER

Amniotic Fluid Embolism

Taru Chhaya

INTRODUCTION

Amniotic fluid embolism (AFE) is one of the most sudden and dangerous emergencies in obstetrics. It usually begins without warning and causes rapid collapse of the heart and lungs, followed by a severe bleeding disorder. Earlier, AFE was believed to occur because amniotic fluid physically blocked the mother's lungs. Today, we understand that AFE behaves more like a severe allergic or immune reaction triggered when certain substances from the amniotic fluid enter the mother's circulation.

Even with modern obstetric and intensive care, AFE continues to cause high maternal morbidity and mortality. Early recognition, quick resuscitation, and well-coordinated teamwork are key to saving lives.

EPIDEMIOLOGY: HOW COMMON AND HOW SERIOUS?

AFE is rare, affecting *approximately 1-12 women per 100,000 deliveries*, depending on the region and reporting methods. Mortality can range from *20 to 60%*. Those who survive often face complications such as:

- Brain injury due to lack of oxygen
- Multi-organ failure
- Severe postpartum hemorrhage requiring massive transfusion or surgery

AFE remains a major cause of direct maternal death worldwide, reminding us that every delivery unit must be prepared for rare but catastrophic emergencies.

EVOLUTION OF UNDERSTANDING

Old theory: A physical embolism of fetal cells blocking pulmonary vessels.

Modern understanding: Anaphylactoid syndrome of pregnancy where maternal immune and inflammatory mechanisms trigger:

- Complement activation
- Mast cell release
- Potent vasoactive mediators

Flowchart 1: Pathophysiology of AFE.

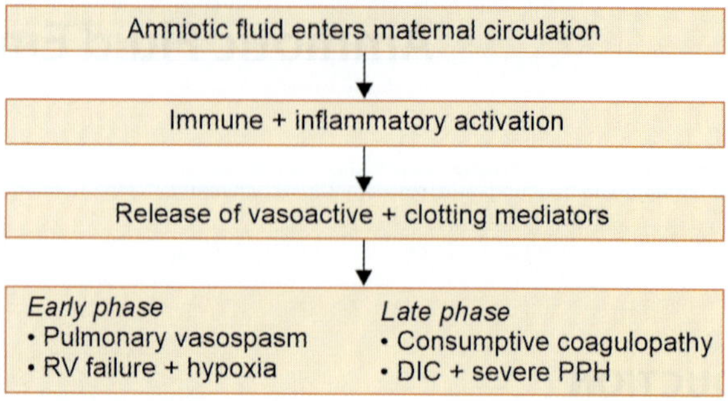

■ PATHOPHYSIOLOGY

See **Flowchart 1**.

■ RISK FACTORS

Although unpredictable, AFE is more frequently reported with:

- Advanced maternal age
- Multiparity
- Placenta previa, abruption, placenta accreta spectrum
- Induction or augmentation of labor
- Operative vaginal delivery
- Cesarean section
- Preeclampsia/eclampsia

However, many women have no risk factors, so vigilance is needed in all labor settings. Rare associations include uterine trauma and second-trimester procedures.

■ CLINICAL PRESENTATION

Classic Triad

AFE typically presents suddenly during labor, soon after delivery, or following an intervention.

The classic triad includes:

1. *Respiratory distress and hypoxia*—sudden dyspnea, cyanosis, drop in oxygen saturation
2. *Cardiovascular collapse*—hypotension, arrhythmias, PEA, or cardiac arrest
3. *Coagulopathy/DIC and severe hemorrhage*—bleeding from puncture sites, uterine atony, uncontrollable postpartum hemorrhage

AFE may start with *cardiorespiratory collapse* or sometimes show *hemorrhage as the first sign.*

Flowchart 2: Diagnosis of AFE.

Sudden cardiorespiratory collapse during labor/postpartum

↓

Check for acute hypoxia (SpO_2 drop, cyanosis, ABG)

↓

Check for coagulopathy/severe PPH (DIC profile)

↓

Exclude other causes (PE, MI, septic shock, anesthesia)

↓

If all above present → clinical diagnosis of AFE

DIAGNOSIS (FLOWCHART 2) CLINICAL AND EXCLUSION-BASED

AFE diagnostic flowchart (Clark criteria).

INVESTIGATIONS

- CBC
- *ABG:* Severe hypoxemia, metabolic acidosis
- *Echo:* Right ventricular failure, pulmonary hypertension
- *Coagulation profile:* Fibrinogen <200 mg/dL, prolonged PT/APTT, thrombocytopenia
- Emerging tests like serum tryptase and complement levels are still research-based.

MANAGEMENT

AFE Response Bundle

No specific cure exists. Management is *supportive, aggressive, and team-based.*

- *Immediate resuscitative measures*:
  - Call the obstetric emergency response team and activate the "Code Blue."
  - Ensure airway patency; provide 100% oxygen and initiate early intubation.
  - Begin high-quality CPR if cardiac arrest occurs, focusing on early chest compressions.
  - Left lateral tilt to reduce aortocaval compression.
- Hemodynamic support:
  - Rapid infusion of IV crystalloids and colloids, Vasopressors (e.g., noradrenaline) to maintain perfusion.
  - Inotropes such as dobutamine for right ventricular failure.

- Continuous cardiac monitoring with frequent reassessment.

3. *Correction of coagulopathy*:
    - AFE-induced consumptive coagulopathy requires immediate activation of a massive transfusion protocol (MTP)
    - Balanced transfusion with PRBC, FFP, and platelets in a 1:1:1 ratio.
    - Early administration of cryoprecipitate to maintain fibrinogen above 200 mg/dL.
    - Tranexamic acid if within 3 hours of hemorrhage onset.
    - Use of TEG/ROTEM for targeted correction of clotting deficits and to minimize transfuse ion delays.
    - Surgical interventions, such as B-Lynch sutures, uterine tamponade balloon, or hysterectomy, may be required in refractory hemorrhage.
4. *Delivery in undelivered mothers*: If cardiac arrest occurs in a pregnant woman beyond 24 weeks, perimortem cesarean delivery within 4 minutes is recommended to relieve aortocaval compression, improve maternal resuscitation effectiveness, and optimize neonatal outcomes.
5. *Rapid recognition checklist (for labor room wall):*

AFE should be suspected if:

- Sudden collapse during labor or just after delivery
- Sudden breathlessness + hypoxia
- Cardiovascular shock or arrest
- Bleeding + clotting disorder (DIC)
  Act immediately, do not wait for tests **(Flowchart 3)**.

RECENT ADVANCES

- *ECMO (VA-ECMO)* for refractory cardiac/respiratory failure shows improved outcomes in specialized centers
- *Recombinant factor VIIa* may benefit uncontrollable bleeding
- Wider use of *TEG/ROTEM* allows more precise transfusion
- *Obstetric early-warning tools* enable earlier detection
- *AFE registries and foundations* are improving global reporting and management protocols

PROGNOSIS

Survival has improved in well-equipped centers with rapid response capabilities.

However:

- Brain injury risk increases with delayed resuscitation
- Neonatal outcomes depend on timing of mother's collapse
- Long-term multidisciplinary follow-up is often required

Flowchart 3: Management of AFE.

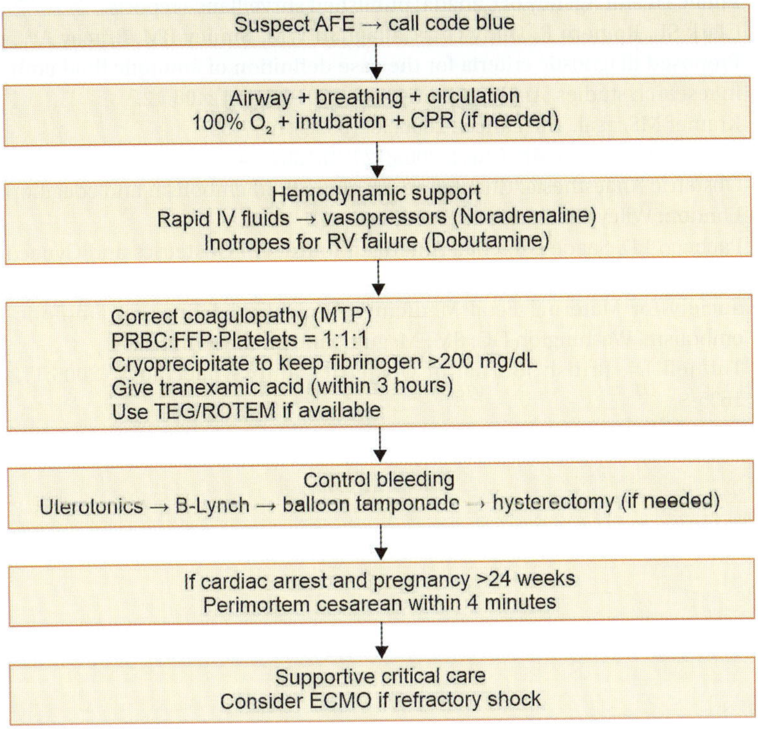

FINAL INSIGHTS

1. AFE is a rare but dramatic emergency requiring immediate recognition and team action.
2. Understanding its immune-mediated mechanism helps improve management.
3. Rapid, protocol-driven resuscitation saves lives.
4. Newer modalities such as ECMO, early fibrinogen replacement, and early-warning tools are promising.
5. Education, reporting, and strengthening preparedness—especially in low-resource settings—are essential.

AFE is ultimately a *test of how quickly and effectively an obstetric team can work together during a crisis.*

SUGGESTED READING

1. AFE Foundation. International Registry Reports. Wisconsin, USA: AFE Foundation; periodically updated reports.
2. Benson MD. Obstetrical & Gynecological Survey. 2007;62(6):377-88.

3. Canadian Perinatal Surveillance System. Maternal mortality reports. Ottawa: Public Health Agency of Canada; published surveillance reports.
4. Clark SL, Romero R, Dildy GA, Callaghan WM, Smiley RM, Bracey AW, et al. Proposed diagnostic criteria for the case definition of amniotic fluid embolism in research studies. Am J Obstet Gynecol. 2016;215(4):408-12.
5. Kramer MS, et al. The Lancet. 2006;368(9535):1447-55.
6. Moore J, Baldisseri MR. Chest. 2005;127(3):1384-94.
7. Obstetric Anaesthesia. Chapter on amniotic fluid embolism and coagulopathy. London: Wiley-Blackwell; latest edition.
8. Pacheco LD, Saade GR, et al. American Journal of Obstetrics and Gynecology. 2018;219(3):B2-B10.
9. Society for Maternal-Fetal Medicine. Clinical guidelines on amniotic fluid embolism. Washington DC: SMFM; guideline publications.
10. Tuffnell DJ. British Journal of Obstetrics and Gynaecology. 2005;112(12): 1625-9.

7 CHAPTER

Acute Abdomen in Pregnancy

S Arulkumaran

INTRODUCTION

Acute abdomen is an emergency. Early diagnosis and management of acute abdominal pain in pregnancy is essential to avoid complications but it can pause difficulties. The pain may be related to pregnancy complications (e.g., ectopic pregnancy, abortion, abruption), that due to problems of the reproductive tract (red degeneration of fibroid, torsion of adnexa) or nonreproductive tract intra-abdominal pathology (urinary infection, renal stone, appendicitis). It is often difficult to differentiate between gynecological, nongynecological, and pregnancy-related causes of abdominal pain. Some of the routine investigations and procedures carry a risk to the fetus such as radiation. This needs to be balanced against the risk of delayed diagnosis and treatment which would be harmful to both mother and/or fetus. Ultrasound scans and X-rays to visualize intraabdominal pathology can pose difficulty with interpretation as the fetal structures may overlap the abdominal pathology (e.g., visualization of a renal stone). Hematological and biochemical parameters may be elevated due to pregnancy related physiological changes rather than due to the pathology. Pain from retroperitoneal structures may be difficult to localize due to the shielding by the uterus and broad ligament. The treatment may be difficult as certain drugs are contraindicated in pregnancy as it may affect the fetus (e.g., indomethacin for pain relief may close the patent ductus, cause pulmonary arterial vasospasm causing pulmonary hypertension or cause renal arterial vasospasm causing oligohydramnios). Doxycycline is contraindicated due to permanent discoloration of baby's teeth; streptomycin use can cause nerve conduction deafness. Surgery may be difficult due to the distended uterus preventing direct approach to an organ. This chapter provides a brief description of various conditions that can cause an acute abdomen, its investigation and management.

ACUTE ABDOMEN: PREGNANCY RELATED (<24 WEEKS)

Miscarriage

Can be associated with lower abdominal dull ache to severe continuous or colicky pain. Vaginal bleeding is present in most cases. Positive urine pregnancy test, pelvic examination, and USS are helpful in diagnosis. Management can be conservative, medical or surgical. A closed cervix, presence of fetal heart on US and doubling of β-hCG every 2 days (in 80%) and increasing progesterone suggests threatened miscarriage and the need for conservative management. Incomplete expulsion of products of conception (incomplete), products in cervical canal (inevitable) and absent FH after 6 weeks and collapsed sac (missed miscarriage) suggests unsuccessful pregnancy and the need for discussion with the woman to opt for expectant, medical (misoprostol 400 μg) or surgical (suction evacuation) therapy.

Ectopic Pregnancy

Presents usually with unilateral lower abdominal pain at <12 weeks of gestation. Associated with brownish vaginal bleeding. Shoulder tip pain is suggestive of hemoperitoneum (bleeding ectopic). Serum hCG does not double every 48 hours in 80%, USS, and laparoscopy are diagnostic. Ultrasound has specific features as shown in the **Figure 1** (empty uterus, adnexal mass, Bagel sign).

The management can be conservative (expectant), medical (IM methotrexate) or surgical by laparoscopy or laparotomy to perform salpingectomy or salpingotomy. The method of treatment depends on the

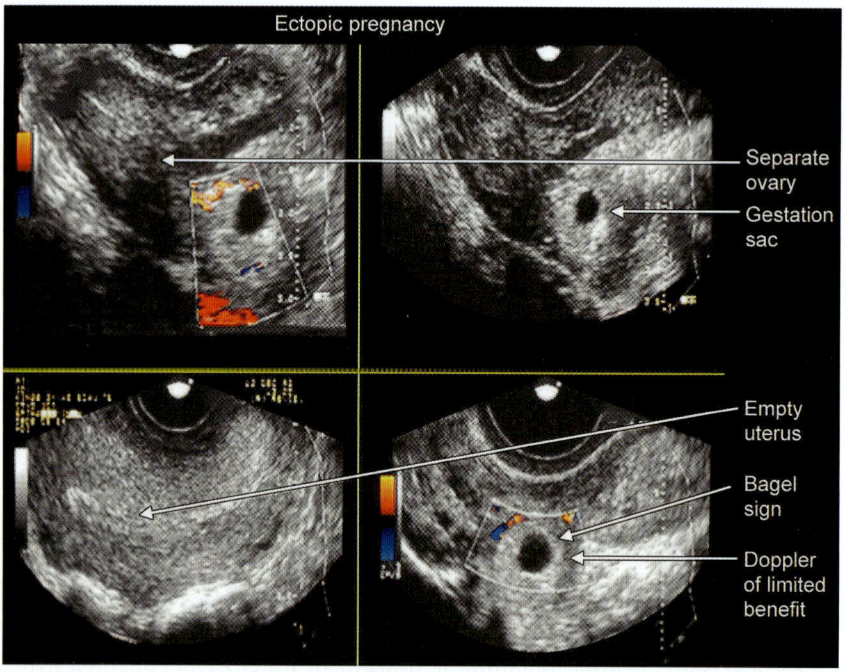

Fig. 1: Ultrasound signs of ectopic pregnancy.

symptoms and signs (pale, pulse, BP), period of gestation, the level of hCG, rate of increase of hCG, presence of FHR.

ACUTE ABDOMEN: PREGNANCY RELATED (>24 WEEKS)

Placental Abruption

Placenta separates partly or completely from uterus before delivery of fetus. This occurs in 0.5% of pregnancies. Blood accumulates behind placenta in uterine cavity or is lost through cervix. Blood seeping into the myometrium causes localized severe pain and tenderness and causes uterine irritability with frequent contractions. Abruption could be concealed: no external bleeding evident (<20%) or revealed with vaginal bleeding emerging via the cervix or mixed where some blood is retained retro placentally and some expelled via the cervix.

Usually presents with abdominal pain of sudden onset, which is continuous in nature unlike intermittent like uterine contractions and may be very severe causing the woman to be pale and faint. Posterior placentas may give rise to severe backache. Diagnosis is made clinically. Ultrasound helps to confirm fetal well-being and exclude placenta previa.

It is safe to admit all women with vaginal bleeding or unexplained abdominal pain and immediately reassure fetal well-being with CTG and to arrange USS as soon as possible to obtain additional information.

IV access with 14 G-orange canula (infuses 240 mL/min or 16 G canula (180 mL/min should be established and bloods sent for Hb, cross match and if clotting defect is suspected for coagulation studies. With massive obstetric hemorrhage, signs are out of proportion to visible blood loss. If fetal distress or maternal compromise, resuscitate and deliver.

Clinically the uterus is tender on palpation. Polysystolic low amplitude uterine contractions suggest blood seeping into the myometrium and causing uterine irritability. At times this could cause fetal compromise exacerbated by the extent of placental separation. Uterus may become "woody hard" and up to 50% may progress into established labor.

Bleeding is very variable, often dark. With increased bleeding, maternal signs of shock will be evident with increasing pulse rate and lowering of BP out of proportion to the revealed bleeding. Fetal distress is common and needs prompt intervention and any delay may result in fetal death.

Uterine Rupture

This usually occurs during labor but has been reported antenatally. Risk factors include previous CS or other uterine surgery; congenital abnormalities of the uterus and induction or augmentation of labor with oxytocin or use of prostaglandins; failure to recognize obstructed labor. The woman presents with acute abdominal pain and tenderness over site of previous uterine scar;

Acute Cholecystitis

This is the second most common surgical condition in pregnancy. Progesterone diminishes smooth muscle tone and predisposes to cholestasis leading to gallstone formation. The incidence of gallstones is 7% in nulliparous and 19% in multiparous women. The incidence of acute cholecystitis is 1–8:10,000 pregnancies. The patient presents with colicky epigastric/right upper quadrant pain, nausea, and vomiting; Murphy's sign may be positive in acute cholecystitis; jaundice indicates obstruction of the common bile duct. Signs of systemic infection of fever and tachycardia may be present. Investigations include FBC, LFTs, CRP (WCC and alkaline phosphatase are increased in pregnancy); increased bilirubin helps to identify patients with concomitant biliary tree obstruction. USS of the biliary tract may demonstrate calculi or a dilated biliary tree. Conservative approach is the most common management with analgesics, antiemetics, hydration and antibiotics.

Cholecystectomy preferably by laparoscopic approach may be indicated in patients with recurrent biliary colic, acute cholecystitis, and obstructive cholelithiasis. This is usually done after delivery of the baby.

Pancreatitis

This occurs more frequently in the 3rd trimester and immediate postpartum period. It can occur in early pregnancy associated with gallstones. Although rare, it is more common in pregnancy than in non-pregnant women of a similar age. The incidence is 1:5,000 pregnancies. Known risk factors are gallstone disease, high alcohol intake and hyperlipidemia.

Common presentation is nausea, vomiting and epigastric pain radiating to the back. Pain is exacerbated by lying flat and relieved by leaning forward serum amylase and lipase levels would be elevated. US examination helps to establish presence of gallstones. Conservative treatment is the mainstay with IV fluids, electrolyte replacement, parenteral analgesics, e.g., morphine (pethidine is contraindicated); resting the bowel with or without nasogastric suction. Early surgical intervention is recommended for gallstone pancreatitis in all trimesters as >70% of patients will relapse before delivery. Laparoscopic or open cholecystectomy can be performed based on the situation. Endoscopic retrograde cholangiopancreatography (ERCP) has a limited role in pregnancy because of radiation exposure to the fetus. If pancreatitis is severe, care in high dependency unit or intensive care unit is preferable due to the need for close frequent observation, careful correction of electrolytes and parenteral pain relief.

FINAL INSIGHTS

All obstetricians should have the knowledge and the clinical acumen to diagnose and manage an acute abdomen.

Clear history taking, attention to the general appearance of the patient, focus on vital parameters, eliciting signs on abdominal and vaginal examination should reveal the diagnosis in most cases.

Hematological, biochemical, X-ray, and ultrasound examination aids in the confirmation of the diagnosis.

Multidisciplinary consultation and care is essential for management of nonpregnancy-related causes that are from the gastrointestinal or renal systems.

Early diagnosis and management will help to reduce adverse outcomes to the mother or fetus.

SUGGESTED READING

1. Royal College of Obstetricians and Gynaecologists. (2022). Diagnosis and management of ectopic pregnancy. [online] Available from https://www.rcog.org.uk/guidance/browse-all-guidance/green-top-guidelines/diagnosis-and-management-of-ectopic-pregnancy-green-top-guideline-no-21/?_gl=1*hqn1n*_up*MQ..*_gs*MQ..&gclid=CjwKCAiA_orJBhBNEiwABkdmjIgBFRZ-53jrG8l-iHPqgjw809CdtBsnpz95DctAcVAAmLbL_srRcxoCCxcQAvD_BwE&gbraid=0AAAAADtSVW5LgVQZQfFhVo-97ispRw62b. [Last accessed January, 2026].
2. Royal College of Obstetricians and Gynaecologists. Early pregnancy loss management. [online] Available from https://www.rcog.org.uk/guidance/browse-all-guidance/green-top-guidelines/early-pregnancy-loss-management-green-top-guideline-no-25/. [Last accessed January, 2026].
3. Sarah Li, Arijit Biswas. Antepartum haemorrhage. In: Arulkumaran S (Ed). Best Practice in Labour and Delivery, 3rd edition. Cambridge: Cambridge University Press; 2025. pp. 172-83.
4. Sekharan PK, Radhadevi VP. Rupture of the uterus. In: Arulkumaran S (Ed). Best Practice in Labour and Delivery, 3rd edition. Cambridge: Cambridge University Press; 2025. pp. 331-42.
5. Zachariah SK, Fenn M, Jacob K, Arthungal SA, Zachariah SA. Management of acute abdomen in pregnancy; current perspectives. Int J Womens Health. 2019;11:119-34.

8 CHAPTER

Transfusion Protocol

Basab Mukherjee

INTRODUCTION

A blood transfusion remains one of the most critical interventions in obstetrics and gynecology. This is especially where catastrophic hemorrhage is sudden as seen during emergencies. Despite advances in healthcare, hemorrhage continues to be a leading cause of preventable maternal morbidity and mortality. This is particularly relevant in low-resource settings such as India.

Transfusion practices in obstetrics must account for the physiological adaptations of pregnancy, i.e., increased cardiac output, expanded plasma volume, and an altered coagulation profile. A structured rational transfusion protocol depends upon the clinical judgement, aims in reducing delays and minimizes inappropriate transfusions. A harmonious communication between obstetricians, anesthetists, intensivists, blood bank officers and hematologists is essential for hassle free services. All obstetricians should have detailed knowledge in decision-making for transfusions, component therapy, and monitoring. Massive transfusion principles **(Box 1)** demand both clinical acumen and system-based teamwork which involves treating the cause of bleeding while simultaneously resuscitating. Procedural, surgical and pharmacological interventions must run parallel to transfusion decisions.

BOX 1: Principles of transfusion in obstetrics.

- Transfuse is directed to restore and maintain the oxygen-carrying capacity
- Component therapy is the standard of care, with targeted correction of red cell deficits, coagulation factor depletion and thrombocytopenia
- Serial assessment is mandatory, as the clinical scenario with obstetric hemorrhage is dynamic and has potential to rapidly deteriorate
- Anticipation is the key and all high-risk women likely to need transfusions should be identified in advance, ideally with blood arranged beforehand
- Request for the least amount of blood or components guided by clinical parameters, estimated blood loss and laboratory indicators
- Multidisciplinary action and timely activation of massive transfusion protocols significantly improve outcomes

BLOOD AND BLOOD COMPONENTS USED IN OBSTETRIC TRANSFUSION

Blood transfusion today is mainly component based which ensures that deficiencies are corrected precisely.

- Plasma
- Packed red blood cells (PRBCs)
- White blood cells
- Platelets
- Fresh frozen plasma (FFP)/cryoprecipitate/fibrinogen concentrate
- Specific clotting factors VII, VIII, XIII, and von Willebrand factor
- Granulocytes
- Albumin
- Immunoglobulins

Whole blood is rarely used today and usually reserved for situations where component therapy is unavailable. A clear understanding of the utility of each component allows for a targeted, rational and safe transfusion.

DECISION TO TRANSFUSE

Acute Blood Loss

In acute obstetric hemorrhage, when it comes to management, the clinical condition supersedes the hemoglobin levels. This is because Hb values lag behind the true circulating loss and take time to be reflected in tests. Clinical parameters include hemodynamic instability, tachycardia, hypotension, narrow pulse pressure, and shock index >1. Evidence of inadequate perfusion include altered mental status, cold extremities and oliguria. Even if Hb is normal or unavailable, transfusion must be initiated if shock is present.

Typical Thresholds

- Hb < 7 g/dL in stable antenatal patients
- Hb < 8 g/dL in laboring/postpartum patients or those undergoing surgery
- Hb < 9 g/dL in women with cardiac disease

Platelets

Transfuse platelets when:

- <50,000/μL with active bleeding or before surgery
- <75,000/μL prior to cesarean in preeclampsia
- <100,000/μL in DIC with FFP (15–20 mL/kg)
- INR or PT/aPTT > 1.5× normal
- Active bleeding with suspected coagulopathy
- Replacement during massive transfusion

Fibrinogen Replacement

- Hypofibrinogenemia is an early marker of severe obstetric hemorrhage.
- Transfuse when fibrinogen < 2 g/L (200 mg/dL).

MASSIVE TRANSFUSION IN OBSTETRICS

Massive transfusion (MT) is defined as ≥4 units of PRBCs in 1 hour or ≥10 units within 24 hours or transfusion required to replace >1 blood volume in 24 hours or any transfusion given for persistent hemorrhagic shock requiring balanced component therapy.

The Obstetric Massive Transfusion Protocol (MTP) aims to replace red cells, coagulation factors, and platelets in ratios approximating 1:1:1. Once triggered, the blood bank prepares predefined packs and coordinates rapid delivery

Goals during MT include:

- Maintaining Hb 8–10 g/dL
- Platelets > 75,000/μL
- INR < 1.5
- Fibrinogen > 2 g/L

The protocol **(Box 2)** must be activated early before coagulopathy becomes irreversible.

Monitoring during and after transfusion is continuous, structured, multidisciplinary.

Important Factors: Pretransfusion

- Verify patient identity, note component type, Rh compatibility, expiry date.
- Baseline vitals—blood pressure, pulse, respiratory rate, temperature, SpO_2.
- Establish large-bore IV access; ensure availability of warming devices.
- Document indication and obtain informed consent whenever feasible.

BOX 2: Protocols for massive transfusion.

During transfusion:

- Observe closely for first 15 minutes (highest risk for acute reactions)
- Monitor vitals at 15 minutes, 30 minutes and every 30 minutes thereafter
- Monitor the respiratory status for early signs of TRALI or TACO
- Urine output (target >30 mL/h)
- Uterine tone to check and excessive vaginal bleeding

Laboratory monitoring (every 30–60 minutes in PPH):

- Hb and hematocrit
- Platelet count
- PT/INR/aPTT/fibrinogen
- Serum electrolytes (calcium especially)
- Lactate and base deficit when ICU monitoring available

Post-transfusion

- Reassess the vital parameters and establish clinical safety
- Document the volume and type of blood components administered
- Monitor for delayed reactions (fever, jaundice, dyspnea, etc.)
- Arrange for follow-up CBC and coagulation studies

MANAGEMENT OF OBSTETRIC HEMORRHAGE USING TRANSFUSION PROTOCOLS

Management Integrates Transfusion with Obstetric Interventions

- Immediate measures are crucial
- Activate hemorrhage protocol
- Call senior obstetrician, anesthetist, and blood bank
- Start crystalloids while preparing for blood components
- Begin uterine massage and uterotonics
- Decision for early transfusion
- Start intervention not waiting for the laboratory confirmation
- PRBCs are started if shock indicators appear
- Simultaneously prepare FFP, cryoprecipitate, and platelets

Component Therapy Targets

- Restore intravascular volume and oxygen transport (PRBCs)
- Correct coagulopathy (FFP)
- Maintain adequate clot formation (platelets + cryoprecipitate)

Ongoing Assessment

- Re-evaluate every 5–10 minutes
- Ensure warming to prevent hypothermia-induced coagulopathy
- Avoid overtransfusion that may cause TACO
- *Escalation if bleeding persists*: Surgical step-up like compression sutures, stepwise devascularization, hysterectomy if needed
- Radiological interventions (whenever available)
- Transfer to HDU/ICU if needed

TRANSFUSION REACTIONS: RECOGNITION AND MANAGEMENT

- A clear and rapid response to transfusion reactions is essential
- The acute hemolytic reaction involves fever, rigors, back pain, and hemoglobinuria. Intervention would be to stop transfusion, maintain urine output, notify the blood bank not to reuse. For febrile nonhemolytic

reaction like mild fever it is advised to pause the transfusion and give antipyretics.

- Allergic or anaphylactic reaction may range from urticaria to airway compromise. Management involves antihistamines or adrenaline depending on the severity.

TRALI stands for *Transfusion-Related Acute Lung Injury*, a serious and potentially fatal complication of blood transfusions that causes sudden respiratory distress. It occurs when antibodies in the donor's blood trigger an immune response in the recipient, leading to fluid build-up in the lungs, i.e., pulmonary oedema. Symptoms include shortness of breath, fever, and cyanosis, and they typically develop during or within six hours of the transfusion. Ventilation support is needed.

TACO typically stands for *Transfusion-Associated Circulatory Overload*, which is a condition where the heart and circulatory system are overwhelmed by the volume of blood transfusion.

Documentation of reactions is mandatory for quality assurance.

FINAL INSIGHTS

A structured transfusion protocol is indispensable for obstetric and gynecological practice, especially where hemorrhage is rapidly progressive and unpredictable. Protocol-driven transfusion aligned with WHO, RCOG, NICE, and ACOG guidelines strengthen clinical decision-making, reduce avoidable delays, and improve maternal outcomes.

For postgraduate trainees, understanding component therapy, recognizing early signs of decompensation, activating massive transfusion protocols promptly and adhering to rigorous monitoring standards are crucial competencies. In India, where hemorrhage still remains a major contributor to maternal mortality, a disciplined application of transfusion protocols is not merely a clinical skill but it is a professional responsibility.

SUGGESTED READING

1. American College of Obstetricians and Gynecologists. Postpartum hemorrhage. Practice Bulletin No. 183. Obstet Gynecol. 2017;130:e168-e186.
2. Collins PW, Lilley G, Bruynseels D, et al. Fibrinogen concentrate in the management of obstetric hemorrhage. Obstet Gynecol. 2014;124(2 Pt 1):261-8.
3. Federation of Obstetric and Gynaecological Societies of India (FOGSI). Good clinical practice recommendations on postpartum hemorrhage and blood transfusion. Mumbai: FOGSI; latest edition.
4. Indian Council of Medical Research. National Guidelines on Blood Transfusion services. New Delhi: ICMR; latest edition.
5. Levy JH, Goodnough LT. How I use fibrinogen replacement therapy in acquired bleeding. Blood. 2015;125(9):1387-93.

6. Mavrides E, Allard S, Chandraharan E, et al. On behalf of the RCOG. Prevention and management of postpartum haemorrhage. BJOG. 2016;124:e106-e149.
7. Ministry of Health and Family Welfare. National blood transfusion services guidelines. Government of India; latest revision.
8. National Institute for Health and Care Excellence. Blood transfusion. NICE Guideline NG24. London: NICE; 2015 (updated 2021).
9. Pavord S, Maybury H. How I treat postpartum hemorrhage. Blood. 2015;125(18):2759-70.
10. Royal College of Obstetricians and Gynaecologists. Blood transfusion in obstetrics. Green-top Guideline No. 47. London: RCOG; 2015 (updated editions available).
11. Shander A, Hofmann A, Isbister J, Van Aken H. Patient blood management—the new frontier. Best Pract Res Clin Anaesthesiol. 2013;27(1):5-10.
12. World Health Organization. WHO recommendations for the prevention and treatment of postpartum haemorrhage. Geneva: World Health Organization; 2012.

9 CHAPTER

Uterine Rupture

Jupirika E Pyrbot

INTRODUCTION

Uterine rupture is a rare but life-threatening obstetric emergency. The incidence of uterine rupture in pregnant patient differs in a scarred and unscarred uterus, with an overall increase incidence in both categories in recent years. Uterine rupture occurs in around 0.2–1% pregnancies with previous one cesarean section and the incidence increases as the number of repeat cesarean deliveries rises. Uterine rupture in an unscarred uterus is much rarer although the incidence may vary both in developed and in developing countries. It is estimated to occur in 1 in 10,000 to 1 in 25,000 pregnancies. The risk of maternal morbidity and mortality is higher in rupture of an unscarred uterus.

ETIOLOGY AND RISK FACTORS

Risk of rupture in scarred uterus:

- Previous uterine rupture
- Previous hysterotomy that involved the upper uterus (e.g., classical incision, high vertical incision, inverted T or J incision)
- Labor, induction, cervical ripening with prostaglandins
- Increasing maternal age
- Birth weight >4,000 grams
- Interdelivery interval less than approximately 18 months (and particularly <6 months)
- More than one previous caesarean birth
- Gestational age ≥41 weeks

A prior vaginal delivery, either before or after the prior caesarean birth, reduces the risk of uterine rupture and improves the likelihood of a successful VBAC.

Risk of rupture, in unscared uterus which may be interdependent:

- Exposure to uterotonic drugs
- High parity
- Short interpregnancy interval
- Prolonged labor

- Uterine anomaly (septate uterus, bicornuate uterus, etc.)
- Uterine overdistension in conditions such as macrosomia, multiple gestation
- Dystocia.
- Placenta accreta spectrum
- Trauma resulting from obstetric maneuver (high forceps, internal or external cephalic version, fundal pressure as well as external physical trauma

STRATEGIES TO REDUCE RISK

Antepartum Imaging

The residual myometrial thickness (RMT) can be measured as early as the first trimester. A 2D or 3D transvaginal ultrasound is typically used to measure the thinnest part of the cesarean scar. The bladder can be partially filled to delineate the serosal lining clearly. A sagittal plane is obtained to identify the uterine niche. The RMT is measured from the tip (deepest point) of the niche in the myometrium to the outer serosal layer. Multiple measurements (typically three) are taken and the smallest value is recorded. Near term, a transabdominal ultrasonography with a partially filled bladder is used to evaluate the scar and measure the RMT. However, available data are limited, as some studies have demonstrated that RMT values may change throughout pregnancy. For this reason, a cutoff value of <2.5 mm near term is commonly used by most authors to predict an increased risk of uterine rupture or dehiscence. The measurement of RMT, along with the adjacent myometrial thickness can assist clinician in counseling patient regarding their individualized risk.

Interpregnancy Imaging

A transvaginal ultrasound performed in a nonpregnant uterus for any gynecological indication can be used to assess cesarean scar integrity. The scar is evaluated in terms of thickness (RMT), any defect: a V or U-shaped defect (niches), and tissue homogeneity. A cesarean scar is considered to be of good quality if the residual myometrial thickness (RMT) is ≥3.5 mm, the myometrium appears smooth and uniform without any defects or ballooning (isthmoceles) and Doppler ultrasound demonstrates good vascularity. Hysteroscopy is used to confirm the diagnoses. Symptomatic isthmoceles can be repaired either laparoscopically or vaginally, with good outcomes in terms of symptom relief. However, routine repair of asymptomatic niches is not recommended. Data on successful vaginal birth after cesarean (VBAC) following isthmocele repair are limited, although subsequent pregnancies and planned cesarean deliveries have been reported.

Obstetric maneuvers and instrumentation should be carried out with caution: External cephalic version or internal cephalic version for malpresentation should be performed cautiously. Instrumental delivery should be performed after proper assessment and feasibility. Fundal pressure applied to a gravid uterus during labor should be avoided.

Use of Uterotonic Agents

Close monitoring of the progress of labor and fetal heart rate with timely obstetric intervention. The use of uterotonics in a grand multiparous or scarred uterus requires careful and continuous monitoring.

Cesarean Delivery

Ensure that the facility is capable for performing immediate cesarean delivery or arranging prompt referral in cases of prolonged labor or arrest of labor.

CLINICAL MANIFESTATION

A sudden change in the pattern of the fetal heart rate may occur, presenting as either a Category II or Category III FHR pattern. In some cases, uterine rupture can lead to the rapid development of severe fetal compromise or even immediate fetal death (intrauterine demise). Thus, it is recommended that the fetal heart rate should be continuously monitored in women undergoing TOLAC.

There may be a change in the pattern of uterine contractions or a complete cessation of contractions. On examination, uterine tenderness may be present, along with changes in the uterine contour. In some cases, the fetus may even be palpated separately from the uterine cavity. On tocodynamometer, findings such as the "staircase sign" may be observed characterized by a gradual decrease in the amplitude of successive uterine contractions.

On Vaginal Examination

Vaginal bleeding may be present, but not in all cases. At times, the bleeding may be minimal, or there may be no vaginal bleeding at all despite significant intra-abdominal hemorrhage. When uterine rupture occurs, the fetus may retract into the abdominal cavity, leading to a loss of station of the presenting part

Uterine rupture may extend into the bladder. In cases of prolonged or obstructed labor, the fetus and uterus can exert direct pressure on a distended bladder, potentially causing bladder laceration and resulting in hematuria.

Intra-abdominal hemorrhage can cause rapid deterioration of the patient's hemodynamic status, potentially leading to hemorrhagic shock

Postpartum

In postpartum patients, occult uterine rupture that occurred during birth is characterized by pain and persistent vaginal bleeding despite use of uterotonic agents. Hematuria may occur if the rupture extends into the bladder.

■ DIAGNOSIS

In a patient presenting with the classic signs—severe abdominal pain, vaginal bleeding, hemodynamic instability, fetal bradycardia or demise, loss of station of the presenting part, and loss of uterine contour—a clinical diagnosis of uterine rupture should be strongly suspected, especially in cases of prolonged labor or during a trial of labor after cesarean (TOLAC). Diagnosis should be based on clinical suspicion, and immediate intervention should be initiated without waiting for radiological confirmation.

■ DIFFERENTIAL DIAGNOSIS

Placental Abruption

Placental abruption has characteristics similar to uterine rupture; however, abruption is associated with increased uterine activity. Additionally, there is no loss of uterine contour and no loss of station of the presenting part.

Intra-abdominal Bleeding

From rupture of a viscus or any major vessel can cause hemodynamic instability in a pregnant woman and may mimic the presentation of uterine rupture.

Placenta Previa

Vaginal bleeding with hemodynamic instability. Can present with rupture signs if complicated with placenta accreta spectrum.

Postpartum Differential Diagnosis

Postpartum hemorrhage that does not respond to uterotonics may require surgical exploration. Following vaginal birth, the presence of severe abdominal pain, vaginal bleeding, and shock may indicate the need for intervention, with radiological confirmation considered if necessary.

■ MANAGEMENT

Immediate Maternal Resuscitation

Patients who are hemodynamically unstable should be given crystalloid, blood, and blood components as they are being prepared for an urgent cesarean section or exploratory laparotomy.

Inform Anesthesia and Pediatrics

General anesthesia is preferred over neuraxial anesthesia, as maternal hypovolemia, potential coagulopathy, and acute fetal compromise are contraindications to neuraxial techniques. Paediatric staff should be alerted in case newborn resuscitation becomes necessary.

Laparotomy

The choice of abdominal incision depends on the operating surgeon, with both midline and transverse incisions being appropriate. Some clinicians prefer a midline incision when hemoperitoneum is suspected, as it allows better exposure of the uterine fundus and adjacent abdominal structures. In contrast, a Pfannenstiel incision provides good access primarily to the lower uterine segment and pelvis.

The fetus is extracted using conventional maneuvers; however, delivery may be challenging if fetal parts have extruded through the site of uterine rupture.

SURGICAL INTERVENTION: HYSTERECTOMY VERSUS REPAIR

Various factors have to be taken into consideration before proceeding toward hysterectomy. The patient's parity and desire for future pregnancy. The extent of uterine damage from the rupture and whether its repairable. The patient's intraoperative hemodynamic and anesthetic stability. The skill of the surgeon for repairing a complicated rupture.

The uterine defect should be repaired in two or three layers using absorbable sutures, similar to the closure of a standard hysterotomy. The use of a single-layer interlocking closure versus a double-layer continuous closure remains a subject of debate. Regardless of the technique chosen, the primary objective is to achieve secure tissue approximation and adequate hemostasis. Medial uterine ruptures that do not compromise the adnexal vasculature are generally amenable to primary closure. Conversely, lateral or markedly extensive ruptures may necessitate ligation of the adnexal vessels and often culminate in hysterectomy. When the defect involves the bladder, or when there is any concern for potential ureteral injury during the laceration or subsequent repair, early involvement of a urologic surgeon is recommended.

MANAGEMENT OF COMPLICATIONS

Atony

Uterine atony may be encountered in uterine rupture which may cause persistent bleeding and should be managed using standard methods, uterotonic agents, hemostatic sutures, and intrauterine balloon tamponade.

When postpartum hemorrhage remains unresponsive to comprehensive medical and surgical management, an obstetric hysterectomy may ultimately be required.

Bladder Trauma

Uterine rupture can result in bladder injury. Intraoperative consultation with a urologic surgeon is recommended. Intraoperative instillation of methylene blue will help identify smaller rents on the bladder. Large anterior ruptures extending into the bladder are typically repaired in two layers, followed by urethral and/or suprapubic catheter placement for up to 14 days. Ureteral injuries though rarer, will require stenting and follow up. Maintaining continuous bladder drainage postoperatively in the setting of suspected bladder injury or obstructed labor supports recovery of contused, devitalized bladder tissue and reduces the risk of vesicovaginal fistula.

Pelvic Organ Injury

Injuries to blood vessels or other pelvic organs should be repaired using standard surgical techniques. Intraoperative consultation with an experienced pelvic, vascular, or general surgeon is advised as needed.

Placenta Accreta Spectrum

Uterine rupture may be associated with placenta accreta spectrum and should be managed according to established protocols for this condition.

■ OUTCOME

Maternal Mortality

The 2010 National Institutes of Health (NIH) Consensus Development Conference on vaginal birth after cesarean reported no cases of maternal death directly attributed to uterine rupture. Maternal mortality from uterine rupture varies widely, ranging from 1–10% or higher in developing countries, compared with approximately 0.1% for rupture of a previous cesarean scar in developed countries. Rupture of an unscarred uterus is associated with a higher risk of poor maternal outcomes than rupture of a scarred uterus.

Morbidity

The two major morbidities associated with uterine rupture are the transfusion of packed red blood cells and the need for hysterectomy. Hysterectomy carries additional risks, including operative injuries such as urinary tract or bowel lacerations, the requirement for blood transfusion, and postoperative infections.

Perinatal Mortality and Morbidity

The perinatal mortality rate associated with uterine rupture ranges from 5% to 26% in case series. Death is most likely when placental separation or fetal extrusion occurs. Even with prompt intervention following uterine rupture, severe neonatal acidosis and associated morbidity or mortality may not always be prevented.

Risk of Recurrent Rupture

Trial of labor after cesarean (TOLAC) should not be offered to patients with a history of prior uterine rupture due to the very high risk of recurrence. The location of the initial rupture is important, ruptures that occur outside the lower uterine segment carry a higher risk of recurrence. Recurrent rupture can occur as early as the second trimester and is difficult to predict.

Timing of Subsequent Pregnancy and Delivery

A short interpregnancy interval increases the risk of uterine rupture in the next pregnancy. Therefore, women planning another pregnancy are advised to maintain a minimum interpregnancy interval of at least 18 months. Elective LSCS in such cases is generally scheduled between 36 and 38 weeks of gestation, although the timing may vary based on the site of the previous rupture. Earlier delivery may be necessary in cases of upper-segment rupture.

Scar Assessment in Future Pregnancies

Scar thickness, integrity, and the presence of an isthmocele can be assessed using transvaginal ultrasound in subsequent pregnancies. A scar demonstrating adequate residual myometrial thickness and good perfusion on Doppler is generally reassuring and associated with a lower risk of rupture. However, it is important to recognize that uterine rupture has occurred even in women with a normal lower uterine segment thickness on antepartum assessment.

UTERINE DEHISCENCE

Uterine dehiscence is an incomplete, clinically silent separation of the uterine wall that typically does not result in significant maternal or neonatal morbidity but may increase the risk of uterine rupture. Most cases are identified incidentally during repeat cesarean delivery, although some can be detected on prenatal ultrasound.

When uterine dehiscence is identified near term, performing a repeat cesarean delivery before the onset of labor is generally considered the safest strategy to prevent progression to complete rupture. When detected remote from term, case reports have described successful outcomes with expectant management involving close surveillance and early delivery if clinically indicated. As no standardized management protocol exists for pregnancies with a thin uterine scar, patients should be thoroughly counseled about the potential maternal and fetal risks that may occur.

FINAL INSIGHT

Uterine rupture is a rare but life-threatening obstetric emergency. Patients undergoing TOLAC must be monitored carefully. All laboring patients receiving uterotonics should be closely monitored, with prompt readiness for surgical intervention whenever there is any deviation in the duration or progress of labor. Uterine rupture can occur at any gestational age; therefore, clinicians must always maintain a high index of suspicion. Timely and appropriate intervention can significantly reduce maternal morbidity and mortality associated with uterine rupture.

SUGGESTED READING

1. Al-Zirqi I, Stray-Pedersen B, Forsén L, Daltveit AK, Vangen S. Uterine rupture: trends over 40 years. BJOG. 2016;123:780-7.
2. Cheung VY. Sonographic measurement of the lower uterine segment thickness: is it truly predictive of uterine rupture? J Obstet Gynaecol Can. 2008;30: 148-51.
3. Chibber R, El-Saleh E, Al Fadhli R, Al Jassar W, Al Harmi J. Uterine rupture and subsequent pregnancy outcome—how safe is it? A 25-year study. J Matern Fetal Neonatal Med. 2010;23:421.
4. Dow M, Wax JR, Pinette MG, Blackstone J, Cartin A. Third-trimester uterine rupture without previous cesarean: a case series and review of the literature. Am J Perinatol. 2009;26:739-44.
5. Gibbins KJ, Weber T, Holmgren CM, Porter TF, Varner MW, Manuck TA. Maternal and fetal morbidity associated with uterine rupture of the unscarred uterus. Am J Obstet Gynecol. 2015;213:382.e1-6.
6. Guise JM, Eden K, Emeis C, Denman MA, Marshall N, Fu RR, et al. Vaginal birth after cesarean: new insights. Evid Rep Technol Assess (Full Rep) 2010;(191):1-397.
7. Hornemann A, Bohlmann MK, Diedrich K, Kavallaris A, Kehl S, Kelling K, et al. Spontaneous uterine rupture at the 21st week of gestation caused by placenta percreta. Arch Gynecol Obstet. 2011;284:875-8.
8. Hunter TJ, Maouris P, Dickinson JE. Prenatal detection and conservative management of a partial fundal uterine dehiscence. Fetal Diagn Ther. 2009;25(1):123-6.
9. Jastrow N, Chaillet N, Roberge S, Morency AM, Lacasse Y, Bujold E. et al. Sonographic lower uterine segment thickness and risk of uterine scar defect: a systematic review. J Obstet Gynaecol Can. 2010;32:321-7.
10. Jastrow N, Demers S, Chaillet N, Girard M, Gauthier RJ, Pasquier JC, et al. Lower uterine segment thickness to prevent uterine rupture and adverse perinatal outcomes: a multicenter prospective study. Am J Obstet Gynecol. 2016;215:604. e1-e6.

11. Jozwiak M, Bloemenkamp KW, Kelly AJ, Mol BW, Irion O, Boulvain M. Mechanical methods for induction of labour. Cochrane Database Syst Rev. 2012;(3):CD001233.
12. Kaczmarczyk M, Sparén P, Terry P, Cnattingius S. Risk factors for uterine rupture and neonatal consequences of uterine rupture: a population-based study of successive pregnancies in Sweden. BJOG. 2007;114:1208-14.
13. Klemm P, Koehler C, Mangler M, Schneider U, Schneider A. Laparoscopic and vaginal repair of uterine scar dehiscence following cesarean section as detected by ultrasound. J Perinat Med. 2005;33:324-31.
14. Martínez-Garza PA, Robles-Landa LP, Roca-Cabrera M, Visag-Castillo VJ, Reyes-Espejel L, García-Vivanco D. Spontaneous uterine rupture: report of two cases. Cir Cir. 2012;80:81-5.
15. Matsuo K, Scanlon JT, Atlas RO, Kopelman JN. Staircase sign: a newly described uterine contraction pattern seen in rupture of unscarred gravid uterus. J Obstet Gynaecol Res. 2008;34:100.
16. National Institutes of Health Consensus Development Conference Panel. National Institutes of Health Consensus Development conference statement: vaginal birth after cesarean: new insights March 8-10, 2010. Obstet Gynecol. 2010;115:1279-95.
17. Osser OV, Jokubkiene L, Valentin L. High prevalence of defects in Cesarean section scars at transvaginal ultrasound examination. Ultrasound Obstet Gynecol. 2009;34:90.
18. Ozdemir I, Yucel N, Yucel O. Rupture of the pregnant uterus: a 9-year review. Arch Gynecol Obstet. 2005;272:229-31.
19. Ridgeway JJ, Weyrich DL, Benedetti TJ. Fetal heart rate changes associated with uterine rupture. Obstet Gynecol. 2004;103:506.
20. Timor-Tritsch IE, Monteagudo A, Calì G, Kaelin Agten A, Palacios-Jaraquemada JM, D'Antonio F. Hidden in plain sight: role of residual myometrial thickness to predict outcome of Cesarean scar pregnancy. Ultrasound Obstet Gynecol. 2023;62:624-32.
21. Usta IM, Hamdi MA, Musa AA, Nassar AH. Pregnancy outcome in patients with previous uterine rupture. Acta Obstet Gynecol Scand. 2007;86:172-6.
22. Wylie BJ, Gilbert S, Landon MB, Spong CY, Rouse DJ, Leveno KJ, et al. Comparison of transverse and vertical skin incision for emergency cesarean delivery. Obstet Gynecol. 2010;115:1134-40.
23. Yang B. Bladder rupture associated with uterine rupture at delivery. Int Urogynecol J. 2011;22:625-7.

10 CHAPTER

Umbilical Cord Prolapse

Biswajyoti Guha

INTRODUCTION

Umbilical cord prolapse is a rare but potentially life-threatening obstetric emergency that requires immediate recognition and swift intervention to reduce perinatal morbidity and mortality. This condition occurs when the umbilical cord descends through the cervix into the birth canal ahead of or alongside the presenting fetal part after the rupture of membranes. Because the cord can easily be compressed between the fetus and the maternal pelvis, rapid diagnosis and appropriate management are crucial to prevent compromised blood flow, hypoxia, or fetal demise.

INCIDENCE

Umbilical cord prolapse is relatively uncommon, with observed incidence rates ranging from 0.1 to 0.9% of all births. Although some studies indicate that the incidence has remained constant over the past century, others attribute a slight decline to decreasing rates of grand multiparity. Occult prolapse, in which the cord lies beside but not beyond the presenting part, is often underdiagnosed; thus, the true incidence may be higher than reported.

RISK FACTORS

Most risk factors for umbilical cord prolapse relate to situations in which the presenting fetal part is not well engaged in the maternal pelvis. Common risk factors include fetal malpresentation such as breech or transverse lies, prematurity, low birth weight, multiple gestations, and polyhydramnios. Maternal factors such as grand multiparity, uterine anomalies, and fibroids may also predispose to prolapse. To reduce incidence, women with abnormal lie after 37 weeks should be counseled regarding admission and advised to seek immediate care if labor or membrane rupture occurs. Fetal factors include excessively long umbilical cord length, marginal cord insertion, and male fetal sex.

Iatrogenic factors can contribute to some cases, especially when obstetric procedures are performed while the presenting part remains high. These include artificial rupture of membranes (amniotomy), induction of labor,

ROLE OF SIMULATION TRAINING

Simulation-based team training plays an important role in improving outcomes. Studies show that regular emergency drills reduce diagnosis-to-delivery intervals and enhance communication, coordination, and procedural efficiency among obstetric staff. Incorporating such training into routine hospital preparedness enhances readiness for managing this unpredictable emergency.

FINAL INSIGHTS

Umbilical cord prolapse remains a critical obstetric emergency that demands rapid recognition and immediate intervention. Although rare, the condition carries significant risk to the fetus due to potential oxygen deprivation. Identifying risk factors, maintaining high suspicion in cases of fetal heart rate abnormalities, and ensuring timely, effective management are key to optimizing outcomes. Advances in obstetric care, including improved surveillance, rapid cesarean delivery capability, and simulation training, have contributed to significantly improved perinatal survival. Ultimately, successful management relies on swift clinical action, effective teamwork, and adherence to established emergency protocols to safeguard maternal and fetal well-being.

SUGGESTED READING

1. Boyle JJ, Katz VL. Umbilical cord prolapse in current obstetric practice. J Obstet Gynaecol. 2005;25(4):303-8.
2. Gibbons C, O'Herlihy C, Murphy JF. A review of umbilical cord prolapse. Eur J Obstet Gynecol Reprod Biol. 2014;175:100-5.
3. Lin MG. Umbilical cord prolapse. Obstet Gynecol Surv. 2006;61(4):269-277.
4. Royal College of Obstetricians and Gynaecologists (RCOG). Umbilical Cord Prolapse. Green-top Guideline No. 50. London: RCOG; 2014.

11 CHAPTER

Trauma and the Unborn

Preeti Sharma

INTRODUCTION

Trauma during pregnancy presents a complex emergency involving two interconnected patients—the mother and the fetus. Trauma is the leading nonobstetric cause of maternal mortality and a major cause of fetal loss. Even mild trauma can cause placental abruption, fetal distress, or preterm labor due to the unique physiological changes of pregnancy. Approximately 6–8% of pregnant women experience some form of trauma, most commonly from road traffic accidents (RTAs), falls, burns, and intimate partner violence (IPV). The concept of "double jeopardy" reflects the dual vulnerability and the need for rapid, multidisciplinary intervention.

TYPES OF TRAUMA IN PREGNANCY

Blunt trauma: The most common mechanism (≈90%), caused by RTAs, falls, or assault.

Penetrating trauma: Stab or gunshot injuries; the fetus is often injured before the mother due to uterine exposure.

Burns: Maternal mortality rises sharply when >50% TBSA is involved, resulting in fetal mortality near 100%.

Chemical/electrical trauma: Rare but associated with systemic toxicity.

Intimate partner violence: Often underreported; linked to miscarriage, fetal growth restriction, and placental abruption.

PHYSIOLOGICAL CHANGES MODIFYING TRAUMA RESPONSE

Cardiovascular: Increased blood volume and cardiac output delay signs of shock. A pregnant woman may lose 30–40% of blood before hypotension develops.

Respiratory: Increased oxygen demand and reduced FRC cause rapid desaturation.

Musculoskeletal: Ligamentous laxity and altered center of gravity increase fall risk.

Uteroplacental circulation: The uterus becomes an exposed organ by 20–24 weeks, increasing risk of abruption.

MATERNAL ASSESSMENT (ABCDE APPROACH)

A—Airway: Soft tissue edema and higher aspiration risk necessitate early airway control.

B—Breathing: Provide 100% oxygen; tilt patient 15° left to avoid aortocaval compression.

C—Circulation: Use two large-bore IV cannulas; use balanced transfusion.

D—Disability: Neurological assessment; differentiate trauma-related seizures from eclampsia.

E—Exposure: Complete examination while preventing hypothermia.

FETAL ASSESSMENT

CTG monitoring: Required ≥4–6 hours for pregnancies ≥24 weeks. Persistent abnormalities require ≥24-hour monitoring.

Ultrasound: Helps assess fetal well-being, placental location, amniotic fluid, and uterine integrity.

Kleihauer-Betke test: Estimates fetomaternal hemorrhage and guides anti-D dosing in Rh-negative mothers.

OBSTETRIC COMPLICATIONS

Placental abruption: The most common cause of fetal death after trauma. Even minor trauma can shear the placenta.

Uterine rupture: Rare but catastrophic; occurs with high-impact trauma, especially in scarred uteri.

Preterm labor: Triggered by stress pathways, abruption, or inflammation.

Fetomaternal hemorrhage: Can lead to fetal anemia or hydrops.

Amniotic fluid embolism: Extremely rare; associated with massive trauma.

MANAGEMENT ALGORITHM

Minor trauma: Observation for 4–6 hours, CTG monitoring, anti-D prophylaxis.

Major trauma: Activate full trauma team, stabilize mother first, continue fetal monitoring, administer steroids <34 weeks.

Indications for emergency delivery:
- Persistent fetal distress
- Uterine rupture
- Severe abruption
- Maternal cardiac arrest (perimortem CS within 4 minutes)

Trauma-specific Situations

RTAs: Leading cause of traumatic fetal loss; proper seat-belt positioning reduces maternal and fetal mortality.

Falls: Common in 3rd trimester due to balance changes.

IPV: A major but hidden cause of recurrent abdominal trauma.

Burns: Fetal survival correlates with maternal TBSA.

Penetrating injuries: High fetal injury due to uterine exposure.

PREVENTION

Patient measures: Proper seat-belt use, fall precautions, reporting IPV early.

Healthcare measures: Trauma drills, rapid referral systems, multidisciplinary care pathways.

FINAL INSIGHTS

Trauma in pregnancy represents a dual-patient emergency. Maternal stabilization is the most important determinant of fetal outcome. Even minor trauma can result in serious fetal harm, making thorough evaluation essential **(Table 1)**. Early CTG monitoring, timely imaging, laboratory evaluation, and coordinated care significantly reduce preventable morbidity and mortality **(Table 2)**. Prevention through education, IPV screening, and safe transport practices is vital.

TABLE 1: Physiological changes affecting trauma.

System	*Pregnancy change*	*Impact on trauma*
Cardiovascular	↑ blood volume, ↑ CO	Delayed shock detection
Respiratory	↓ FRC, ↑ O_2 need	Rapid desaturation
GI	Organ displacement	Atypical injury pattern
Uterus	Exposed organ	↑ Abruption risk
Hematologic	Hypercoagulable	↑ VTE risk

TABLE 2: Red flags after trauma.

Red flag	*Action*
Uterine tenderness	24–48 hours monitoring
Vaginal bleeding	USG + laboratories
>4 contractions/h	Assess for abruption
Abnormal CTG	Consider delivery
Maternal instability	ICU transfer

SUGGESTED READING

1. Barraco RD, Chiu WC, Clancy TV, Como JJ, Ebert JB, Hess LW, et al.; EAST Practice Management Guidelines Work Group. Practice management guidelines for the diagnosis and management of injury in the pregnant patient: the EAST Practice Management Guidelines Work Group. J Trauma. 2010;69(1):211-4.
2. El Kady D. Perinatal outcomes after trauma. Clin Obstet Gynecol. 2007;50(3):582-91.
3. Hoffman MK, Sciscione AC. Blunt trauma in pregnancy: maternal and fetal outcomes. Obstet Gynecol. 1997;90(4 Pt 1):544-8.
4. Ikossi DG, Lazar AA, Morabito D, Fildes J, Knudson MM. Profile of mothers at risk: an analysis of injury and pregnancy loss in 1,195 trauma patients. J Am Coll Surg. 2005;200(1):49-56.
5. Jain V, Chari R, Maslovitz S, Farine D, Bujold E, Gagnon R, et al. Guidelines for the Management of a Pregnant Trauma Patient. J Obstet Gynaecol Can. 2015;37(6):553-74.
6. Krulewitch CJ, Pierre-Louis ML, de Leon-Gomez R, Guy R, Green R. Seat belt use during pregnancy: prevalence and patterns among women in the United States. Am J Obstet Gynecol. 2000;182(4):1043–6.
7. Levine AB, Livingston DH, Sperling L, McLellan BA, Shires GT. Trauma during pregnancy: a review of maternal and fetal outcomes. Emerg Med Clin North Am. 1994;12(1):167-99.
8. Mendez-Figueroa H, Dahlke JD, Vrees RA, Rouse DJ. Trauma in pregnancy. Am J Obstet Gynecol. 2013;209(1):1-10.
9. Pearlman MD, Tintinallli JE, Lorenz RP. A prospective controlled study of outcome after trauma during pregnancy. Am J Obstet Gynecol. 1990;162(6): 1502-7.
10. Petrone P, Talving P, Browder T, Teixeira PG, Fisher O, Lozornio A, et al. Abdominal injuries in pregnancy: a 155-month study at two level 1 trauma centers. Injury. 2011;42(1):47-9.

12 CHAPTER

Thyroid Storm

Nidhi Chaturvedi

INTRODUCTION

Thyroid storm, also known as the thyrotoxicosis crisis, is a life-threatening emergency characterized by excess of thyroid hormones leading to multiorgan dysfunction.

It occurs in women with poorly controlled or undiagnosed hyperthyroidism precipitated by an acute event like infection, trauma, surgery, or labor.

Hyperthyroidism in pregnancy has a reported incidence of 0.2%. Common causes include Grave's disease, gestational transient thyrotoxicosis, which are the most common, toxic multinodular goiter, toxic adenoma, pituitary adenoma, struma ovary, and thyroiditis.

Grave's disease is an autoimmune disorder characterized by thyroid receptor antibodies (TRAbs) which bind with the thyroid stimulating hormone (TSH) receptor causing increased amounts of thyroid hormones T3 and T4.

Gestational transient thyrotoxicosis is a unique entity presenting in the first trimester. Rising hCG values stimulate the TSH receptor due to their molecular analogy resulting in increased levels of thyroid hormones. It can also be associated with molar pregnancy or hyperemesis gravidarum or multiple pregnancy with raised levels of hCG. However, typical signs and symptoms of hyperthyroidism are not seen, and it resolves in a few weeks requiring no treatment.

Currently all countries recommend risk-based screening of thyroid function in pregnant women. Indian Thyroid Society recommends universal screening. This will help in detection of cases of both subclinical and overt thyroid dysfunction and their timely management.

Unless diagnosed preconceptionally and adequately treated, hyperthyroidism can cause severe complications, the most serious being the thyroid storm.

Thyroid storm is a rare endocrine emergency resulting from sudden and excessive amounts of thyroid hormone activity. It is characterized by a hypermetabolic state with rapid deterioration leading to nonobstetric cause of maternal mortality. In pregnancy, most cases occur due to one of the preexisting underlying causes of hyperthyroidism, most commonly

Grave's disease. Precipitating factors include infection, stress, trauma, or sudden withdrawal of antithyroid drugs. In pregnancy, preeclampsia, induction of labor, cesarean section, and pregnancy itself can precipitate thyroid storm.

CLINICAL FEATURES

Clinically woman exhibits signs of high metabolic rate and increased oxygen demand with high fever >103°F, tachycardia >140/minute, high blood pressure due to preeclampsia complicating pregnancy, signs of heart failure(shortness of breath and edema), nausea, vomiting, diarrhea, dehydration, agitation, anxiety, seizures, and confusion. Lack of treatment for hyperthyroidism or family history of hyperthyroidism may help in diagnosis.

LABORATORY STUDIES

Measurement of TSH with free/total T4 may be done. Reference ranges of these hormones in pregnancy are different and should be used. If total T4 value specific to trimester not available, a value equal to 1.5 times the value in nonpregnant woman should be used. However, it has been found that actual hormone levels in thyroid storms may not be different from that in hyperthyroidism. TRAbs help in the diagnosis of Grave's disease.

COMPLICATIONS

Physiological increase in the blood volume and cardiac output may predispose the pregnant woman to cardiac failure and arrythmias. Higher incidence of cardiomyopathy is seen in pregnant women with thyroid storm. Fluid and electrolyte disturbances due to gastrointestinal symptoms and cardiac failure may cause kidney and liver damage. Obstetric complications include preeclampsia, abruption, preterm birth, low birth weight, fetal thyroid dysfunction, and poor maternal and fetal outcome.

Thyroid storm is a clinical diagnosis. Scoring systems like Burch-Wartofsky Point Scale (BWPS) and the Japan Thyroid Association (JTA) criteria are available for assessment of severity, but not validated in pregnancy.

DIFFERENTIAL DIAGNOSIS

- Sepsis
- Preeclampsia
- HELLP
- Heart failure
- Psychosis
- Pheochromocytoma

MANAGEMENT

According to the American Thyroid Association guidelines, management is based on the principles of:

- Reducing the amount of thyroid hormones both synthesis and secretion—antithyroid drugs
- Preventing the conversion of T4 to active T3, thus reducing the peripheral effects—PTU and glucocorticoids
- Supportive therapy
- Management of the inciting event
- Management of pregnancy

General Measures

These women are managed in intensive care settings (ICU)

- Crystalloids with electrolyte correction
- Antipyretics and cooling
- Find underlying cause
- Avoid delivery

Antithyroid Drugs

PTU is preferred first line drug as it reduces the peripheral conversion of T4 to T3. Loading dose of 500–1,000 mg followed by 250 mg 4 hourly is given per oral (PO), per rectal (PR) or by nasogastric tube (NGT).

Methimazole may be given if PTU not available (20 mg 6 hourly). After the storm subsides, PTU may be continued in the first trimester as methimazole can cause serious congenital malformations such as aplasia cutis and choanal atresia.

Methimazole is continued after the woman improves, in the 2nd and 3rd trimesters.

β-blockers

Propanol is a nonselective β-blocker, administered in a dose of 60–80 mg every 4 hourly to control heart rate. Preferred drug by the American Thyroid Association (ATA) as it inhibits conversion of T4 to T3, and its dose can be adjusted. Esmolol is B1 selective and has a short half-life so preferred by the Japan Thyroid Association (JTA) as beta blockers can cause cardiogenic shock in pregnancy. Atenolol can cause FGR and not given.

Iodide-SSKI (saturated solution of potassium iodide) administered 1hour after first dose of PTU (5 drops every 6 hours) blocks thyroid hormone synthesis.

Hydrocortisone helps prevent conversion of T4 to T3. It also helps tide over the stressful event by supporting the adrenals and autoimmunity due to Grave's disease.

Dose: 300 mg IV loading dose then 100 mg 8 hourly.
Antibiotics if infection precipitated the storm.
Cholestyramine in refractory cases.
Thyroidectomy if compression of trachea, preferably in 2nd trimester.

FINAL INSIGHTS

- Thyroid storm is a rare but potentially life-threatening complication in pregnancy.
- Diagnosis is clinical with symptoms hyperpyrexia, severe tachycardia, heart failure, gastrointestinal and neurological disturbances.
- History of hyperthyroidism with improper treatment may help in recognition.
- Reference values of TSH/T4 in each trimester different from nonpregnant individuals.
- Treatment is prompt and aggressive, done in ICU setting.
- Antithyroid drugs with iodide, beta blockers, and steroids form the mainstay of treatment.
- Delivery should be avoided.
- The Indian Thyroid Society recommends universal screening of thyroid function in all antenatal women.

SUGGESTED READING

1. Akamizu T, Satoh T, Isozaki O, Suzuki A, Wakino S, Iburi T, et al. Diagnostic criteria, clinical features, and incidence of thyroid storm based on nationwide surveys. Thyroid. 2012;22(7):661-79.
2. Alexander EK, Pearce EN, Brent GA, Brown RS, Chen H, Dosiou C, et al. 2017 guidelines of the American thyroid association for the diagnosis and management of thyroid disease during pregnancy and the postpartum. Thyroid. 2017;27:315-89.
3. Burch HB, Wartofsky L. Life-threatening thyrotoxicosis. Thyroid storm. Endocrinol Metab Clin North Am. 1993;22(2):263-77.
4. Goldman AM, Mestman JH. Transient non-autoimmune hyperthyroidism of early pregnancy. J Thyroid Res. 2011:2011:142413.
5. Ma Y, Li H, Liu J, Lin X, Liu H. Impending thyroid storm in a pregnant woman with undiagnosed hyperthyroidism. Medicine. 2018;97:e9606-4.
6. Pokhrel B, Aiman W, Bhusal K. Thyroid Storm. Treasure Island (FL): StatPearls Publishing; 2025.
7. Prabawa A, Negara KS. Diagnosis and Comprehensive Management of Thyroid Storm in Pregnancy: A Case Report. Biomed Pharmacol J. 2018;11(3).
8. Rajput R, Bajaj S, Ghosh S, Kalra P, Menon AS, Pillai MG, et al. Thyroid disorders in pregnancy: Consensus statement of Indian Thyroid Society. Thyroid Res Pract. 2021;18:89-110.
9. Satoh T, Isozaki O, Suzuki A, Wakino S, Iburi T, Tsuboi K, et al. 2016 Guidelines for the management of thyroid storm from The Japan Thyroid Association and Japan Endocrine Society (First edition). Endocr J. 2016;63(12):1025-64.

10. Schroeder BM; American College of Obstetricians and Gynecologists. ACOG practice bulletin on thyroid disease in pregnancy. Am Fam Physician. 2002;65(10):2158, 2161-2.
11. Sorah K, Carlson K. Hyperthyroidism in Pregnancy. Treasure Island (FL): StatPearls Publishing; 2025.
12. Sugiyama Y, Tanaka R, Yoshiyama Y, Ichino T, Hishinuma N, Shimizu S, et al. A case of sudden onset of thyroid storm just before cesarean section manifesting congestive heart failure and pulmonary edema. JA Clin Rep. 2017;3(1):20.
13. Thyroid Disease in Pregnancy ACOG Practice Bulletin, Number 223. Obstet Gynecol. 2020;135(6):e261-74.
14. US Food & Drug. (2018). FDA Drug Safety Communication: New Boxed Warning on severe liver injury with propylthiouracil. [online] Available from https://www.fda.gov/drugs/postmarket-drug-safety-information-patients-and-providers/fda-drug-safety-communication-new-boxed-warning-severe-liver-injury-propylthiouracil#aihp. [Last accessed January, 2026].
15. Vadini V, Vasistha P, Shalit A, Maraka S. Thyroid storm in pregnancy: a review. Thyroid Res. 2024;17(1):2.

13 CHAPTER

Preterm Prelabor Rupture of Membranes

Suyoga Panat

INTRODUCTION

The most exciting and nerve wrecking part of pregnancy is labor, but if it happens too early it may be the most scarry thing to experience for any patient, moreover if the membranes rupture prematurely it may become very challenging for the patient as well as treating obstetricians.

Whenever there is rupture of fetal membranes before the onset of labor and before 37 weeks of gestation it is called as PPROM, it leads to one-third cause of premature deliveries and associated perinatal complications.

INCIDENCE

It complicates 8–10% of all pregnancies and due to prematurity, it is responsible for maternal risk of sepsis, as well as neonatal mortality and morbidity including respiratory distress syndrome, ischemic brain damage, necrotizing enterocolitis, retinopathy of prematurity, etc.

There is a period of brief latency from the time of rupture of membranes to delivery. The dilemma is whether to do expectant management or wait for spontaneous labor or to induce it. Secondly, while doing expectant management the risk of infection increases.

MECHANISMS

At term there is collagen remodeling, cellular apoptosis, and it leads to progressive weakening of the membranes. When there is onset of labor, due to the increased intrauterine pressure, there is spontaneous rupture of membranes. PPROM near term may be due to these physiological processes in many of the cases **(Fig. 1)**.

However, in cases where there is PPROM remote from term, certain pathologic processes like infection and inflammation occur, also role of ascending infection seems reasonable as the bacterial proteases can lead to membrane weakening.

There can be a maternal inflammatory response like the production of prostaglandins, cytokines, etc. which can lead to weakening and degradation of the membranes due to the ascending bacterial colonization.

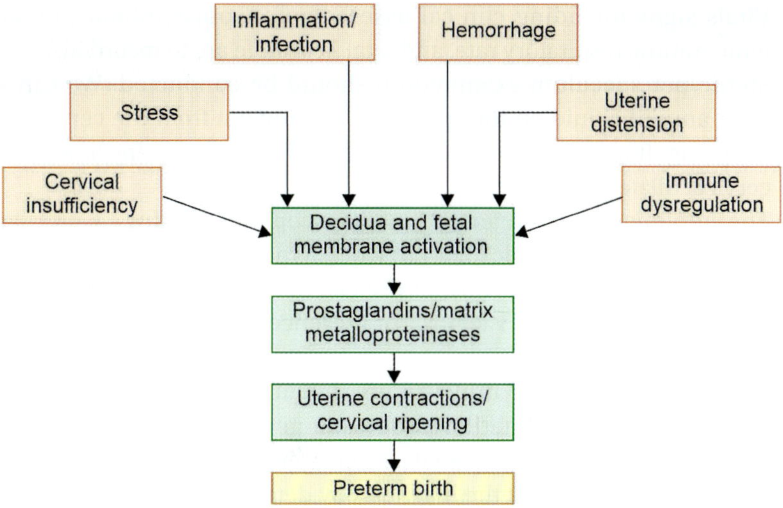

Fig. 1: Factors leading to preterm birth.

CLINICAL RISK FACTORS

- Previous history of PPROM
- Polyhydramnios
- Twin pregnancy
- Bacterial vaginosis
- Urogenital infections
- Uterine bleeding
- Cervical incompetence
- Cervical cerclage
- Procedures like amniocentesis
- Abdominal trauma or history of fall
- Collagen vascular disorders
- Low socioeconomic status
- Maternal malnutrition and anemia
- Cigarette smoking
- Maternal stress can result in hormonal and cytokine activation and preterm contractions leading to prom

There can be genetic predisposition to PPROM may be due to collagen metabolism in certain connective tissue disorders.

The chances of recurrence of PPROM are 16–32%.

DIAGNOSIS AND EVALUATION

Diagnosis depends on history, examination of patient, and appropriate investigations. These are the considerations for initial assessment in PPROM.

- Mostly the patient gives history of excessive watery discharge per vaginum or sometimes just a trickle leaking.

- Vitals signs including clinical assessment of pulse, blood pressure, temperature, respiratory rate, and fetal heart rate are to recorded.
- Sterile per speculum examination should be conducted. We can see clear amniotic fluid on the speculum coming out from the cervix or on coughing. It also helps to rule out any cord prolapse, helps in assessing cervical dilatation.
- The amniotic fluid is subjected for microscopic fern testing.
- The pH of vagina is acidic (3.8–4.5) whereas amniotic fluid is alkaline (pH is 7.1–7.3), so a simple pH paper test can be done. If there is presence of blood, semen, bacterial vaginosis or presence of lubricants, false positive result can occur.
- A high vaginal swab and urine culture should be done.
- Digital vaginal examination should be generally avoided to reduce chorioamnionitis or minimum if patient appears to be in labor.
- Ultrasound can support the diagnosis by determining the amniotic fluid volume. It is also helpful to evaluate the exact gestational age, estimated fetal weight, presentation of fetus and localization of placenta or any evidence of abruption.
- Maternal blood tests including c-reactive protein and white blood cell count should be done.

After the diagnosis and gestational age is confirmed, the neonatal team should be informed and if the neonatal care facilities are inadequate consider in utero transfer to higher center.

CLINICAL COURSE

In 50% of the patients of PPROM delivery occurs within 1 week of membrane rupture whatever may be the clinical presentation.

After the rupture of membranes, the latency is inversely correlated with the gestational age at the time of rupture.

Infrequently the leakage stops and the normal amniotic fluid restoration occurs chorioamnionitis occurs in 15–35% of cases and in 15–25% cases postpartum infection can occur. In 2–5% cases abruption is seen.

PPROM can be managed as inpatient or in selected cases as outpatient department.

When the patient is admitted after confirmation of the diagnosis, monitor maternal uterine activity and clinically assess signed of chorioamnionitis, i.e., fever > 38°C. or 100.4°F with maternal as well as fetal tachycardia and uterine tenderness along with vaginal discharge. WBC count > 16,000/mm^3 is supportive to the clinical findings if antenatal corticosteroids are not administered within 5–7 days.

If these signs are seen, fetal heart rate is nonreassuring, significant vaginal bleeding is seen delivery should be conducted. In the absence of these signs conservative management can be considered. If the patient is stable gestational age is the most important factor in determining the continuation of conservative management.

Prophylactic antibiotic (GBS) prophylaxis should be started. A 7-day antibiotic therapy should be started.

Antibiotic of Choice

- Combination of intravenous ampicillin [2 g 6 hourly) and erythromycin (250 mg 6 hourly) for 48 hours]
- Oral amoxycillin 250 mg thrice a day and erythromycin 250 mg thrice a day

Amoxiclav (amoxycillin and clavulanic acid) is not preferred as it may increase the risk of necrotizing enterocolitis.

Corticosteroids

- Short-term tocolysis can be given in the presence of uterine contractions till the effect of corticosteroid occurs if the gestational age is >34 weeks.
- If administered within 48 hours of birth they are most effective.

Mechanism

Corticosteroids cross the placenta and the amount of surfactant produced by type II pneumocytes when given in divided doses they provide many neonatal benefits. It helps in reducing the risk of respiratory distress syndrome, necrotizing enterocolitis and intraventricular hemorrhage.

Dosage of Corticosteroids

- 4 doses of injection dexamethasone 6 mg 12 hourly intramuscular or
- 2 doses of injection Betnesol 12 mg 24 hours apart intramuscularly.

There is greater reduction of RDS while using betamethasone as compared to dexamethasone.

Rescue dose of corticosteroids can be given in preterm PROM < 34 weeks if the prenatal corticosteroids are given 14 days prior and are at risk of delivery within 7 days.

Magnesium Sulfate

If the gestational age is <30 weeks and delivery seems eminent magnesium sulfate can be started. It significantly reduces the risk of cerebral palsy and gross motor dysfunction.

Magnesium sulfate is a neuroprotector. 4 g intravenous bolus of $MgSO_4$ is given over 20 minutes followed by 1 g intravenous infusion per hour until delivery or for 24 hours whichever is earlier. This is endorsed by RCOG.

SUGGESTED READING

1. Dayal S, Jenkins SM, Hong PL. Preterm and Term Prelabor Rupture of Membranes (PPROM and PROM). Treasure Island (FL): StatPearls Publishing; 2024.
2. Gravett MG, Menon R, Tribe RM, Hezelgrave NL, Kacerovsky M, Soma-Pillay P, et al. Assessment of current biomarkers and interventions to identify and treat women at risk of preterm birth. Front Med (Lausanne). 2024;11:1414428.
3. Layden EA, Thomson A, Owen P, Madhra M, Magowan BA. Clinical Obstetrics and Gynaecology, 5th edition. Amsterdam: Elsevier; 2022.
4. Malhotra N, Garg R, Goyal P. Clinical Protocols in High Risk Pregnancy: A Case-based Approach. New Delhi: Evangel Publishing Pvt. Ltd.; 2025.
5. Prelabor Rupture of Membranes: ACOG Practice Bulletin, Number 217. Obstet Gynecol. 2020;135(3):e80-97.
6. Royal College of Obstetricians and Gynaecologists. Magnesium Sulphate to Prevent Cerebral Palsy following Preterm Birth (Scientific Impact Paper No. 29). London: Royal College of Obstetricians and Gynaecologists; 2011.
7. Saxena P, Nigam A. A Practical Approach to Management of Preterm Labor. New Delhi: Evangel Publishing Pvt. Ltd.; 2019.
8. Spong CY, Lockwood CJ. Queenan's Management of High-Risk Pregnancy: An Evidence-Based Approach, 7th Edition. New Jersey: Wiley; 2023.
9. Ugwumadu L, Ugwumadu A. Preterm Birth. In: Bhide AG, Arulkumaran S, Damania K, Daftary SN, Schubbe AA (Eds). Arias' Practical Guide to High Risk Pregnancy, 6th edition. Amsterdam: Elsevier; 2024.

14 CHAPTER

Diabetic Ketoacidosis in Pregnancy

Poonam Goyal, Pallaavi Goel

INTRODUCTION

Diabetic ketoacidosis (DKA) is a life-threatening metabolic emergency characterized by hyperglycemia, ketosis, and metabolic acidosis. In pregnancy, it is associated with rapid maternal deterioration and acute fetal compromise, with fetal loss rates reported between 10–35%. The physiological changes of pregnancy lower the threshold for DKA, leading to euglycemic DKA where glucose may be only mildly elevated.

As diabetes prevalence rises across India, especially insulin-requiring gestational diabetes, GOI, FOGSI, ACOG, WHO and NICE/RCOG all recommend protocol-driven management to reduce preventable maternal morbidity and fetal death.

Early recognition and immediate emergency management are critical in the labor management.

PATHOPHYSIOLOGY

It is different in pregnancy as it is in itself a "ketogenic stress state" due to several interacting mechanisms:

- Insulin resistance increases from mid-pregnancy due to placental hormones (hPL, progesterone, cortisol, prolactin, growth hormone).
- Rapid lipolysis → excess free fatty acids → accelerated hepatic ketogenesis.
- Physiological respiratory alkalosis reduces buffering capacity → quicker and more severe acidosis.
- Increased GFR and osmotic diuresis → rapid dehydration and electrolyte loss.
- Elevated metabolic demands mean missed insulin or reduced food intake can quickly trigger ketosis.

Even mild stress such as vomiting or infection may precipitate DKA more aggressively than in non-pregnant adults.

FETAL IMPACT

Fetal compromise in DKA results from maternal physiological instability:

- Severe acidemia → fetal myocardial depression

- Reduced uteroplacental perfusion → fetal hypoxia
- Electrolyte shifts (K^+) → arrhythmias
- Hyperosmolarity → fluid imbalance in placenta and fetus

Most fetal heart rate abnormalities improve once maternal metabolic state stabilizes—hence maternal rescue is must for fetal rescue.

COMMON PRECIPITATING FACTORS

Seen frequently in emergency settings:

- *Infections:* UTI, pneumonia, dengue, gastroenteritis
- Missed insulin (cost issues, gaps in care, pump failure, carelessness)
- Vomiting/starvation (including during religious fasts)
- Antenatal corticosteroids for fetal lung maturity
- β-agonist tocolytics
- Undiagnosed Type 1 diabetes presenting acutely
- Poor ANC follow-up due to access and socioeconomic barriers

Every insulin-using pregnant woman should receive written sick-day rules.

CLINICAL PRESENTATION

Symptoms can mimic normal pregnancy:

- Nausea, vomiting, abdominal pain (may be mistaken as labor)
- Polyuria, polydipsia
- Tachypnea/Kussmaul breathing
- Dehydration, tachycardia
- Altered mental state in advanced acidosis

Red flag triad: Vomiting + tachypnea + ketonuria → consider DKA even with near-normal glucose.

DIAGNOSIS IN PREGNANCY

- Diagnostic parameters are given in **Table 1**.
- Assess severity and comorbid conditions for HDU/ICU admission.

TABLE 1: Diagnostic parameters.

Component	*Indicator*
Glucose	Often >200–250 mg/dL (may be normal)
Ketones	Blood β-OHB ≥3 mmol/L or moderate–high urine ketones
pH	<7.30
HCO_3^-	<18 mmol/L
Anion gap	>12

EMERGENCY MANAGEMENT: LABOR WARD/ED

Maternal stabilization first followed by fetal resuscitation.

Follow standard emergency sequence:

ABCDE approach in DKA—stepwise

- A—Airway
  - Check if airway is patent, patient is alert and able to speak
  - Protect airway if drowsy (aspiration risk)
- B—Breathing
  - Assess respiratory rate and pattern (e.g., Kussmaul respiration)
  - Provide oxygen if $SpO_2 < 94\%$ or maternal distress
- C—Circulation
  - Establish IV access
  - Start fluid resuscitation with 0.9% saline
  - Monitor potassium and hemodynamics closely
- D—Disability
  - Assess sensorium (GCS)
  - Check capillary blood glucose immediately
- E—Exposure
  - Complete examination looking for infection, dehydration signs or abdominal tenderness
  - Obstetrics causes

Once mother is stabilized then Fetal assessment is done with USG/Doppler/CTG whatever is indicated.

FLUID REPLACEMENT (CORNERSTONE OF RESCUE)

- *Start 0.9% saline:* 1 L in first hour (15–20 mL/kg)
- Continue 0.9%/0.45% saline 250–500 mL/h (adjust per BP/UOP/Na^+)
- When glucose <180–200 mg/dL → add 5% dextrose
- Avoid fluid overload in cardiac disease or preeclampsia

  Correcting hypovolemia is important for uteroplacental perfusion.

Insulin Therapy—Fixed Rate IV Infusion

- 0.14 units/kg/h continuous IV insulin
- *Target glucose drop:* 50–75 mg/dL/h
- If glucose 200 decrease the infusion rate to 0.02–0.05 per kg/h
- If blood glucose falls add dextrose to avoid hypoglycemia
- Continue until anion gap closes and ketones normalize

Do not stop insulin early—ketones must clear once the DKA is normalized shift the patient subcutaneous insulin.

TABLE 2: Potassium replacement protocol.

K^+ level	*Action*
<3.3 mmol/L	Hold insulin, give K^+ till ≥3.3
3.3–5.3 mmol/L	20–30 mmol KCl per L
>5.3 mmol/L	Recheck hourly

TABLE 3: Parameters for monitoring in emergency.

Parameter	*Frequency*
Capillary glucose	Hourly
Blood ketones	2–4 hourly
Electrolytes + ABG/VBG	2–4 hourly
Strict fluid input/output	Continuous
CTG after viability	Continuous

Potassium Replacement—Lifesaving

- Hypokalemia commonly worsens after insulin **(Table 2)**
- Severe shifts ↑ arrhythmia risk → continuous ECG if K^+ unstable.

Bicarbonate

- Not routinely indicated.
- Consider only if pH <6.9 with hemodynamic compromise and after senior review.

TREAT UNDERLYING CAUSE

- Empirical antibiotics pending cultures if infection
- Stop β-mimetics where possible
- Steroid insulin adjustment—often 20–40% increase
- Review psychosocial barriers to insulin access

MONITORING IN EMERGENCY/LABOR WARD

Parameters for monitoring in emergency are given in **Table 3**.

OBSTETRIC CONSIDERATIONS

- Nonreassuring CTG early in DKA is typically secondary to maternal compromise and improves with correction.
- Avoid immediate delivery unless independent obstetric emergency:
  - Abruption
  - Uterine rupture
  - Fetal bradycardia unresponsive to maternal correction

- If in labor:
  - Continue IV insulin-dextrose protocol
  - Hourly glucose + ketones
- Maintain glucose 90–120 mg/dL
- Discuss delivery timing postrecovery per IUGR, glycemic control, and comorbidities

  Anesthetic implications—correct pH and K^+ before neuraxial block.

COMPLICATIONS

Maternal

- Severe dehydration and shock
- Electrolyte imbalance → arrhythmias
- ARDS and AKI
- Cerebral edema (rare but catastrophic)

Fetal

- Fetal demise
- Hypoxic-ischemic encephalopathy
- Preterm birth and NICU admission

Continuous improvement of maternal metabolic state → best fetal survival.

For prevention preconception optimization with HbA1c <6 we reduce DKA risk. Regular ANC is important watch for FPG < 90 mg/dL, 1-h PPG <140 mg/dL in insulin-requiring GDM and T1/T2DM. We should encourage home ketone monitoring in insulin-dependent women. We can even give her written sick-day rules. Never stop basal insulin.

Hospital Readiness

- Labor ward DKA algorithm poster
- Ketone meters, infusion pumps, and K^+ fluids available
- Regular simulation drills for residents

FINAL INSIGHTS

- DKA in pregnancy is rapid and unforgiving
- Diagnosis requires vigilance for lower-glucose DKA
- Fixed-protocol emergency management improves outcomes
- Treat mother first—fetal restoration usually follows
- Prevention via education, ANC structure, and hospital systems is essential
- Multispecialty care with involvement of diabetologist and pediatrician is the key.

A well-trained team, a clear DKA protocol, and timely action directly reduce maternal and fetal morbidity.

SUGGESTED READING

1. American College of Obstetricians and Gynecologists. ACOG Practice Bulletin No. 201: Pregestational Diabetes Mellitus. Obstet Gynecol. 2018;132(6):e228-48.
2. American Diabetes Association. Standards of Medical Care in Diabetes 2022: Diabetes in Pregnancy. Diabetes Care. 2022;45(Suppl 1):S232-43.
3. Federation of Obstetric and Gynaecological Societies of India (FOGSI). Good Clinical Practice Recommendations–Hyperglycemia in Pregnancy. Mumbai: FOGSI; 2023.
4. Government of India, Ministry of Health and Family Welfare. National Guidelines for Diagnosis and Management of Gestational Diabetes Mellitus. New Delhi: Ministry of Health and Family Welfare; 2014.
5. ICOG–FOGSI. Screening and Management of Hyperglycemia in Pregnancy. Mumbai: FOGSI; 2021.
6. National Institute for Health and Care Excellence. NG3: Diabetes in pregnancy: management from preconception to the postnatal period. London: National Institute for Health and Care Excellence; 2020.
7. World Health Organization. Diagnostic criteria and classification of hyperglycaemia first detected in pregnancy. Geneva: World Health Organization; 2013.

15 CHAPTER

Lessons from Maternal Near Miss

Poonam Joon

INTRODUCTION

Maternal health has long been a sensitive indicator of the performance of any healthcare system. Reducing maternal mortality is the Millennium Development Goal 5. To reach this goal, countries need an accurate picture of the causes and levels of maternal deaths. Maternal mortality (MM) is frequently described as "just the tip of the iceberg" alluding that there is a vast base to the iceberg in the form of maternal near miss (MNM), i.e., maternal morbidity which has remained largely undescribed. It is also assumed to be a better indicator than maternal mortality alone for designing, monitoring, follow-up and evaluation of safe motherhood programs.

WHO established a technical working group of obstetricians, midwives, epidemiologists and public health professionals from developing and developed countries to develop a maternal death classification system. The working group also reached consensus on how to define maternal near miss—"a woman who nearly died but survived a complication that occurred during pregnancy, childbirth or within 42 days of termination of pregnancy".

The global prevalence of maternal near-miss (MNM) is estimated to be around 1.4% (14 per 1,000) live births, though this varies widely by region. The World Health Organization (WHO) has established criteria to identify these events, and studies using the WHO criteria report different rates, for example, a near-miss rate of 20.55 per 1,000 obstetric admissions or 23.85 per 1,000 live births in one study. The incidence of MNM is 11/1,000 live births; the ratio of MNM to maternal deaths is 1.2:1 in another study in Maharashtra.

In 2009, WHO has come up with clinical, laboratory, and management criteria for the identification of these cases **(Table 1)**.

As per the Operational Guidelines Ministry of Health & Family Welfare Government of India, the following criteria (minimum three; one from each category) must be met with for identification of an MNM case:

1. Clinical findings (either symptoms or signs)
2. Investigations
3. Interventions

Or any single criteria which signifies cardiorespiratory collapse.

TABLE 1: Criteria for identification of near miss cases.

Criteria	*Description*	*Advantages*	*Disadvantages*
Clinical criteria related to a specific disease entity	Disease specific definitions used for common conditions and clinical criteria defined for severe morbidity, e.g., preeclampsia is a disease and complications such as eclampsia, renal failure and pulmonary edema identify severe cases	• Easy to interpret; cases can be identified retrospectively • Quality of care of that disease can be identified	• All problems may not be covered • Difficult to define and quantify the condition
Management specific	Management or intervention to disease, e.g., hysterectomy, blood transfusion or admission to ICU	Simple to use in identification of cases	Depends on other variables such as availability of ICU beds, indications for hysterectomy
Organ system dysfunction or failure	Based on the concept that there is a sequence of events leading from good health to death. Death is preceded by organ dysfunction and organ failure. Markers for organ system dysfunction or failure are specified, e.g. jaundice in the presence of preeclampsia	Allows for identification of critically ill women Keeps focus on severe diseases	Dependent on the existence of a minimum level of care including functioning laboratories and basic critical care monitoring

The clinical findings, investigations and interventions have been put under three broad categories **(Annexure 2)**

1. Pregnancy specific obstetric and medical disorders
2. Preexisting disorders aggravated during pregnancy
3. Accidental/incidental disorders in pregnancy

These broader categories have further been segregated under different clinical situations like haemorrhage, sepsis, hypertension, etc.

There are two formats in which the data need to be entered:

1. Facility based Maternal Near Miss Review (FBMNM-R) form—**Annexure 1**
2. MNM-R case register—details of columns to be made in the register—**Annexure 3**

Annexure 2 illustrates the criteria for diagnosing the MNM.

(**Annexure 1, 2, and 3** as in Maternal Near Miss Review December 2014 Operational Guidelines Ministry of Health & Family Welfare Government of India).

Signs of organ dysfunction that follow life-threatening conditions are used to identify maternal near misses so that the same classification of underlying causes is used for both maternal deaths and near miss.

SALIENT FEATURES OF MNM ANALYSIS

MNM cases offer richer and more frequent data than maternal deaths. For every woman who dies, several others experience life-threatening complications. These survivors can share first-hand accounts, allowing clinicians and researchers to trace the sequence of events, delays, and factors that contributed to the critical episode enabling a deeper understanding of preventable causes, identification of modifiable risk factors, continuous monitoring of maternal health services, and timely evaluation of interventions.

The Three-Delay Model remains extremely relevant in explaining the chain of events leading to MNM:

Delay in seeking care: MNM analyses consistently highlight awareness regarding danger signs such as severe bleeding, convulsions, reduced fetal movement, or severe headaches.

Delay in reaching care: Many MNM cases show that even when families decide to seek help, the time taken to reach a tertiary facility can be critical.

Delay in receiving quality care: The third delay is often the most crucial. Shortages of skilled staff, lack of blood products, delayed diagnosis, poor triage, inadequate monitoring, and systemic inefficiencies are common themes emerging from MNM reviews.

Antenatal care remains a powerful preventive tool in early registration, regular monitoring, counseling on danger signs, birth preparedness, and family planning.

Timely recognition and early intervention is one of the most consistent lessons. Early diagnosis and prompt action are the difference between life and death. MNM analyses reveal that structured triage protocols, standardized early-warning score systems (like MEOWS) and simulation-based emergency drills improve response times and reduce complications.

Continuous medical education ensures timely adoption of evidence-based practices. The competence, training, and teamwork of healthcare providers are critical in managing obstetric emergencies

Health system preparedness like timely access to blood and blood products, well-equipped ICUs, functional operation theatres, availability of magnesium sulfate, uterotonics, IV fluids, antibiotics, clear referral protocols, adequate documentation are critical. Stock-outs or equipment malfunction in emergencies can be catastrophic.

Importance of effective communication between healthcare workers (handover protocols), between primary and tertiary centers (referral communication), between providers and patients (explaining danger signs) and within teams during emergencies (closed-loop communication) is crucial.

Respectful maternity care (RMC) is not just ethical, it has survival benefits. Compassionate communication improves cooperation during emergencies.

Social determinants of health play a major role and MNM cases serve as a reminder that maternal health cannot be improved without addressing deeper social determinants like poverty, illiteracy, gender inequality, malnutrition, teenage pregnancies, advanced maternal age and lack of antenatal care

The need for continuous quality improvement as MNM transforms a negative event into an opportunity for systemic learning and better preparedness. Important lessons include establishing Maternal Near Miss review committees, conducting structured root-cause analyses implementing low-cost, high-impact interventions (e.g., PPH kits, checklists) monitoring MNM ratios and severe maternal outcome ratios over time.

Psychological impact as a result of surviving a life-threatening obstetric event often leads to psychological trauma so MNM care must include psychological rehabilitation.

Policy level implications and the way forward as MNM findings emphasize the need for strengthened primary care and midwifery-led units, universal access to emergency obstetric and newborn care (EmONC), incentivizing institutional deliveries, awareness campaigns on danger signs and birth preparedness. These measures can significantly reduce both maternal mortality and severe morbidity.

Maternal near miss cases serve as powerful lens into the functioning of maternal health systems. They offer invaluable lessons such as clinical, administrative, social, and policy-oriented. By examining not only what went wrong but also what went right in saving a woman's life, MNM reviews help create resilient health systems capable of preventing maternal deaths and reducing severe morbidity. Studying maternal near miss shifts the focus from counting deaths to saving lives, reflecting a proactive vision for safer motherhood.

FINAL INSIGHTS

Maternal near-miss cases provide a critical framework for assessing the performance of health systems. Near-miss events occur more frequently and yield equally valuable insights into the pathways leading to severe morbidity and mortality. Survivors share their experiences directly, are less threatening for service providers while offering invaluable insights and realistic evaluation into the systemic gaps. This enables policymakers and practitioners to identify women most at risk of maternal death, guiding allocation of resources to areas of greatest need. Every near-miss should be embraced as an urgent call to action and an opportunity to strengthen the quality of maternal health services.

SUGGESTED READING

1. Kulkarni R, Chauhan S, Fidvi J, Nayak A, Humane A, Mayekar R, et al. Incidence and factors influencing maternal near miss events in tertiary hospitals of Maharashtra, India. Indian J Med Res. 2023;158(1):66-74.
2. Ministry of Health and Family Welfare. Maternal Near Miss Review. New Delhi: Ministry of Health and Family Welfare, Government of India; 2014.
3. Parmar NT, Parmar AG, Mazumdar VS. Incidence of Maternal "Near-Miss" Events in a Tertiary Care Hospital of Central Gujarat, India. J Obstet Gynaecol India. 2016;66(Suppl 1):315-20.
4. Pattinson R, Say L, Souza JP, Broek NV, Rooney C; WHO Working Group on Maternal Mortality and Morbidity Classifications. WHO maternal death and near-miss classifications. Bull World Health Organ. 2009;87(10):734.
5. World Health Organization. Evaluating the quality of care for severe pregnancy complications the WHO near-miss approach for maternal health. Geneva: World Health Organization; 2019.
6. World Health Organization. Report on the World Health Organization Working Group on the Classification of Maternal Deaths and Severe Maternal Morbidities. Geneva: World Health Organization; 2009.

Maternal Near-miss Case Scenarios

Swati Singhal

INTRODUCTION

Maternal mortality, while a critical indicator of a nation's healthcare quality, represents only the "tip of the iceberg" of severe maternal morbidity. For every maternal death, numerous women experience life-threatening complications but survive due to timely intervention and quality care; these are known as "maternal near misses" (MNM). According to the World Health Organization (WHO), a maternal near-miss case is defined as "a woman who nearly died but survived a complication during pregnancy, childbirth or within 42 days of termination of pregnancy" (WHO, 2011). While maternal mortality reviews provide essential insights into failures within health systems, MNM audits offer a complementary lens by examining cases where survival was achieved. These events capture a broader spectrum of morbidity and highlight opportunities for improving clinical care, health system responsiveness, and emergency preparedness.

Globally, MNM indicators have become essential for monitoring quality of obstetric care. For every maternal death, it is estimated that 20–30 women experience a near-miss event. Near-miss case reviews thus provide rich opportunities to identify delays, inadequacies in care, and areas for clinical capacity-building. This chapter presents few representative MNM case scenarios, followed by analytical commentary and discussion of cross-cutting themes.

CASE SCENARIO 1: PLACENTA ACCRETA SPECTRUM (PAS)—A HEMORRHAGE CRISIS

A 32-year-old multiparous woman with two prior cesarean sections presented at 37 weeks with placenta previa. Antenatal imaging suggested possible focal accreta, but limited access to advanced imaging at the district hospital prevented precise assessment. She was referred late to a tertiary care center for delivery.

During cesarean section, torrential hemorrhage occurred immediately upon attempting placental removal. Dense placental invasion into the myometrium and extension toward the bladder indicated placenta increta. A massive transfusion protocol was initiated, and an emergency hysterectomy was performed. The patient required six units of packed red cells, four units of fresh frozen plasma, and two units of platelets. Postoperatively, she was admitted to the ICU for hemodynamic stabilization and extubated on day two. She survived without long-term organ dysfunction. This case met maternal near-miss criteria due to massive hemorrhage, shock, and the requirement for life-saving hysterectomy.

Analysis: Late referral and identification of the condition antenatally worsen the situation.

Positive factor: Immediate activation of the massive transfusion protocol, Successful execution of an emergency cesarean hysterectomy, postoperative ICU admission and stabilization.

Lessons learned: The importance of antenatal diagnosis, pre-operative planning, and the availability of a well-coordinated multidisciplinary team and adequate blood bank support in a tertiary care center cannot be overstated for managing PAS.

CASE SCENARIO 2: HYPERTENSIVE EMERGENCY LEADING TO ECLAMPSIA

A 32-year-old multiparous woman presented at 34 weeks with severe headaches and blurred vision. Blood pressure was 170/112 mm Hg, and she had +++ proteinuria. Although she met criteria for severe preeclampsia, the initial clinician opted to "observe" and postponed magnesium sulfate administration. Four hours later, the patient had a generalized tonic-clonic seizure. She was stabilized with magnesium sulfate, antihypertensives, and emergency delivery. Despite severe metabolic derangement, she recovered after 72 hours in the ICU.

Analysis:
- *Primary cause:* Severe preeclampsia evolving into eclampsia.
- *Contributing factors:* Failure to identify the urgency of severe hypertension.
- Delay in administering magnesium sulfate.

Positive factors:
- Rapid emergency response once seizure occurred.
- Availability of critical care.

Learning points:
- Severe preeclampsia is a medical emergency—magnesium sulfate must be initiated promptly.
- Blood pressure control should begin within 30–60 minutes of identifying severe hypertension.
- Training gaps in recognition of hypertensive emergencies remain a global issue.

5. World Health Organization. Evaluating the quality of care for severe maternal morbidity: the WHO near-miss approach for maternal health. Geneva: World Health Organization; 2011.
6. World Health Organization. Evaluating the Quality of Care for Severe Pregnancy Complications: The WHO Near-Miss Approach for Maternal Health. Geneva: World Health Organization; 2011.
7. World Health Organization. Maternal sepsis. Geneva: World Health Organization; 2025.

17 CHAPTER

Near-miss Navigator: Practical Tips

Mitra Saxena

DEFINITION

A maternal near miss is defined by the World Health Organization as, a woman who survives a severe complication during pregnancy, childbirth, or postpartum period within 42 days, highlighting potential gaps in care.

IMPORTANCE OF IDENTIFYING AND MANAGING MNM CASES

Maternal death is a sentinel event, whereas a maternal near miss event serves as a proxy model for maternal death and provides information to evaluate factors that caused deterioration or steps taken, which saved the patient.

Maternal death reviews are threatening with element of blame game and concealment of facts thereof, for fear of punitive action, whereas maternal near miss reviews are met with more acceptable participation by all the stake holders and serve as a sound basis to formulate policies, guidelines for adopting corrective measures for the three delay model.

The three delay model comprises of Level one—delay in decision to seek care, Level two—delay in reaching care, Level three—delay in receiving adequate health care.

CLASSIFICATION OF NEAR-MISS CASES IN OBSTETRICS

MNM can be classified as:

- Types of near miss cases (e.g., hemorrhage, hypertensive disorders, and sepsis)/nonobstetric reasons for MNM
- Based on severity classification (e.g., mild, moderate, severe)

Some key indicators to watch for:

- Severe postpartum hemorrhage
- Hypertensive disorders
- Sepsis
- Organ dysfunction
    1. Severe maternal complications (e.g., hemorrhage, hypertensive disorders, sepsis) based on specific disease conditions
    2. Clinical criteria (e.g., organ dysfunction respiratory, cardiovascular, and renal)

3. Management based criteria (e.g., ICU admission blood transfusions and emergency surgery)

Hence it is very important to evaluate all maternal near miss cases:

- To highlight areas for improvement in maternal care
- To provide insights into severe maternal morbidity
- To propose strategies for reducing maternal mortality

Government of India has implemented many directives to bring down MMR and MNM ratio.

Reader is advised to refer to mohw.gov.in directives.

WHAT A PRACTICING OBSTETRICIAN-GYNECOLOGIST SHOULD DO? PRACTICAL TIPS

Our basic premise is *predict, prevent, perform, and progressive periodic assessments*

Practical tips: The 4Ps*

Predict (Anticipate)

- *Identify high-risk patients:* Anemia, hypertension, high risk cases to be filtered early
- Recognize early warning signs
- Use risk assessment tools

Prevent (Avoid)

- *Implement evidence-based protocols:* AMTSL/use of magnesium sulfate
- Ensure timely interventions/use of NASG
- Foster a culture of safety

Perform (Manage)

- Effective communication and teamwork/presence of senior obstetrician/multidisciplinary teams when needed
- Timely and appropriate interventions
- Continuous monitoring and support

Progressive Periodic Assessments

- Conduct debriefing sessions
- *Identify gaps in care:* Team readiness and facility preparedness by:
  - Training and response of healthcare providers
    - Preparedness of healthcare facilities
    - Documentation and communication
  - Develop plans to address these gaps

AUDITS

Regular review of near miss cases helps in:

- Analysis of contributing factors
- Recognize areas for improvement
- Develop and implement corrective measures
- Create checklists and protocols to prevent similar incidents
- Implementation of quality improvement measures

FINAL INSIGHTS

A maternal near miss (MNM) case often serves as a wake-up call for healthcare providers, highlighting the thin line between life and death. While it is natural to breathe a sigh of relief when a patient survives a life-threatening complication, it is crucial to harness this experience to improve future care.

FINAL TAKE AWAYS

1. *Use standardized criteria:* Adopt WHO's near miss criteria or adapt local guidelines.
2. *Train healthcare providers:* Educate staff on recognition and documentation.
3. *Monitor high-risk patients:* Closely track patients with preexisting conditions or complications.
4. *Conduct regular audit:* Review cases to identify potential near misses.
5. *Encourage reporting*: Foster a culture of transparency and encourage staff to report cases.
6. *Use triggers:* Identify triggers such as ICU admission, blood transfusion, or emergency surgery.
7. *Collaborate with multidisciplinary teams:* Involve obstetricians, anesthetists, and other specialists in reviews

SUGGESTED READING

1. Mantel GD, Buchmann E, Rees H, Pattinson RC. Severe acute maternal morbidity: a pilot study of a definition for near-miss. BJOG. 1998;105(9): 985-90.
2. Ministry of Health and Family Welfare, Government of India. Guidelines for maternal near-miss review operational framework. New Delhi: Ministry of Health and Family Welfare; 2014.
3. Say L, Souza JP, Pattinson RC. Maternal near miss—towards a standard tool for monitoring quality of maternal health care. Best Pract Res Clin Obstet Gynaecol. 2009;23(3):287-96.
4. World Health Organization. Evaluating the quality of care for severe pregnancy complications: the WHO near-miss approach for maternal health. Geneva: World Health Organization; 2011.

18 CHAPTER

Maternal CPR

Ranju Singh

INTRODUCTION

Cardiac arrest during pregnancy is rare but uniquely challenging because clinicians must simultaneously prioritize maternal survival and consider fetal well-being. Physiological changes of pregnancy, specific causes of arrest (e.g., massive obstetric haemorrhage, amniotic fluid embolism, pulmonary embolus), and the mechanical effects of the gravid uterus require some modifications to standard adult basic and advanced life support (BLS/ALS) algorithms. Recent international resuscitation guidance (AHA/ILCOR/ERC 2025 updates) retains core cardiopulmonary resuscitation (CPR) principles while emphasizing interventions specific to pregnancy, notably continuous left uterine displacement (LUD), early airway management, upper extremity intravenous access above diaphragm, early multidisciplinary team activation, attention to reversible obstetric causes, and timely decision-making about perimortem cesarean delivery (PMCD).

PHYSIOLOGY AND IMPLICATIONS FOR RESUSCITATION

Pregnancy produces important cardiovascular and respiratory changes: Increased cardiac output and blood volume, reduced functional residual capacity, increased oxygen consumption, and upward displacement of the diaphragm from the enlarging uterus. After roughly 20 weeks of gestation (fundus at or above the umbilicus), the gravid uterus can compress the inferior vena cava and aorta when the woman is supine, reducing venous return and cardiac output-aortocaval compression that can worsen coronary and cerebral perfusion during arrest. Awareness of these changes explains why left uterine displacement (LUD) or lateral tilt is a central modification to standard CPR in pregnant patients. Effective resuscitation requires a structured, well-organized approach guided by established protocols to ensure optimal patient outcomes and there is a growing need for standardized training focused on maternal resuscitation. The basic steps to be followed when pregnant woman collapses are discussed here.

Scene Safety and Assess Responsiveness

Approach the patient ensuring scene safety and determine unresponsiveness by tapping the shoulders from the front and calling out loudly: "Are you okay?" The absence of any purposeful response confirms the need for further evaluation.

Call for Help and Activate the Maternal Resuscitation Team

Immediately shout for help. Direct a specific person to call the emergency number like 112 (Emergency Response Support System) or 102 (ambulance service) if outside the hospital or activate the hospital's cardiac arrest/Code Blue system when in the hospital. It is crucial to state clearly: "cardiac arrest in a pregnant woman." This ensures rapid mobilization of key personnel—obstetricians, anesthesiologists, neonatologists, intensivists, nursing staff, and operating room support. Simultaneously request for the AED/defibrillator and maternal cardiac arrest kit. Early team activation is associated with improved maternal and neonatal outcomes. Ensure that you also give relevant location details and do not end the call until instructed.

Check Breathing and Pulse Simultaneously (No More Than 10 Seconds)

Look for normal breathing, agonal breaths are not considered normal breathing. Simultaneously palpate the carotid pulse for 5–10 seconds. If no pulse or no/abnormal breathing (gasps only) is detected, immediately begin CPR. Delays beyond 10 seconds reduce the chance of survival.

Start High-Quality Chest Compressions Immediately

Place hands on the lower half of the sternum and begin compressions at a rate of 100–120/min and depth of 5 6 cm. Allow full chest recoil and minimize interruptions (to <10 seconds). The patient should be on a firm flat surface and hips should be at the level of the patient's chest. High-quality compressions are the single most important determinant of survival and must be prioritized throughout. Rotate compressors every 2 minutes to avoid fatigue. A designated team leader should monitor compression quality continuously.

RELIEVE AORTOCAVAL COMPRESSION: CONTINUOUS MANUAL LEFT UTERINE DISPLACEMENT

If the uterus is at or above the umbilicus (≥20 weeks of gestation), the gravid uterus can compress the inferior vena cava and aorta, compromising venous return and cardiac output. To counter this immediately apply manual left uterine displacement (LUD). An assistant uses both hands to pull the uterus upward and to the left. The LUD is now recommended if there is more than one rescuer, left lateral tilt is to be avoided as it reduces compression quality significantly. Manual LUD must continue uninterrupted throughout CPR.

ATTACH THE AED/DEFIBRILLATOR

As soon as the AED arrives, apply the defibrillation pads without pausing compressions. Use standard pad positions (antero-lateral or antero-posterior). Follow the AED prompts: if shockable rhythm (VF/pVT) → announce "all clear" and deliver shock immediately and resume compressions after the shock delivery. If the rhythm is nonshockable (asystole/pulseless electrical activity) continue CPR and proceed with airway and circulatory interventions. Pregnancy is not a contraindication to defibrillation, and energy doses remain unchanged. Chest compressions should resume immediately after shock delivery without pausing to check for a pulse. Any fetal monitoring devices, whether internal or external, should be removed or disconnected before shock delivery, due to the theoretical risk of shock transmission to the fetus. However, time should not be wasted on removing these devices if it delays defibrillation.

AIRWAY MANAGEMENT AND VENTILATION

Open the airway with the "head tilt and chin lift" maneuver. Give two breaths after every 30 compressions using a pocket mask or bag-mask device with 100% oxygen. Take 1 second each for the inspiration and expiration and look for adequate chest rise as indication for sufficient tidal volume. Given the high risk of rapid desaturation, early advanced airway management is recommended. A second generation supraglottic device (i-gel® and Ambu® Aura-i™) can be easily inserted by the rescuer and used as a definitive airway device. Intubation should only be attempted by the most experienced provider, avoiding delayed oxygenation and with full preparedness for a difficult airway. The Society for Obstetric Anesthesia and Perinatology recommends using a video laryngoscope at the first intubation attempt. Rapid sequence induction is not indicated. Once intubated, maintain continuous compressions, ventilate at 10 breaths/min, and use waveform capnography to confirm and monitor placement.

ESTABLISH VASCULAR ACCESS ABOVE THE DIAPHRAGM

Place intravenous (preferably) or intraosseous access in the upper extremities to ensure drug delivery to the central circulation. Administer medications as per standard ACLS protocols (epinephrine every 3–5 minutes, antiarrhythmics as indicated). Maternal resuscitation always takes priority; fetal medication exposure is secondary.

IDENTIFY AND TREAT REVERSIBLE CAUSES (PREGNANCY-SPECIFIC)

While CPR continues, consider the standard reversible causes (5 H's and 5 T's) and add pregnancy-specific conditions:

- Massive obstetric hemorrhage
- Amniotic fluid embolism
- Pulmonary embolism (thrombotic or air)
- Eclampsia/severe preeclampsia
- Magnesium toxicity
- Uterine rupture
- Cardiomyopathy/peripartum cardiomyopathy.

Treat identified causes simultaneously—activate massive transfusion, administer magnesium antagonist if needed, give thrombolysis where appropriate, and consider extracorporeal membrane oxygenation (ECMO) in advanced centers if there is no return of spontaneous circulation (ROSC).

PREPARE EARLY FOR PERIMORTEM CESAREAN DELIVERY (PMCD)

Current 2025 recommendations reinforce the "4-minute rule": If there is no ROSC by approximately 4 minutes in a patient with uterus ≥20 weeks, initiate PMCD. The aim is to deliver by 5 minutes to improve maternal circulation and optimize fetal salvage. Removing the fetus can improve maternal cardiac output by up to 60% by alleviating aortocaval compression. It also facilitates more effective chest compressions and enhances respiratory mechanics. The PMCD must not be delayed waiting for an operating theatre. The procedure should be performed at the site of arrest, including emergency room or ward, as moving the patient wastes critical time. The PMCD term has now been renamed as resuscitative hysterotomy (RH) in the recent guidelines.

CONTINUE CYCLES OF CPR AND ONGOING MANAGEMENT

Reassess rhythm every 2 minutes. Continue defibrillation if shockable rhythms persist. Adjust airway, ventilation, and circulatory support as needed. Maintain continuous LUD and ensure optimal compression quality. After ROSC, initiate postresuscitation care with attention to hemodynamics, oxygenation, targeted temperature management where appropriate, and preparation for definitive obstetric intervention.

TEAM DYNAMICS, SYSTEMS, AND SIMULATION

Maternal cardiac arrest requires seamless teamwork. Clear role allocation—compressor, airway manager, LUD provider, drug/defibrillator handler, team leader, obstetric surgeon, and neonatal team—prevents duplication and errors. Clear message delivery, closed loop communication, knowledge sharing, summary and evaluation, constructive intervention and mutual respect are the pillars of effective team dynamics that significantly enhance teamwork and contribute to improved patient outcomes. Institutions must maintain:

- A maternal cardiac arrest protocol
- A PMCD equipment kit
- Regular multidisciplinary simulation training
- Mechanisms for post-event debriefing
- Systems-level readiness significantly improves survival and neurological outcomes.

FINAL INSIGHTS

Maternal cardiac arrest is a rare but high-stakes emergency demanding rapid, coordinated, and pregnancy-specific actions. The 2025 guidelines reaffirm that maternal resuscitation is the priority and provide clear direction: begin high-quality compressions immediately, apply continuous left uterine displacement, secure airway and circulation promptly, defibrillate without hesitation, and proceed to perimortem cesarean delivery within 4–5 minutes if no ROSC is achieved. Consistent adherence to these steps, combined with institutional preparedness and multidisciplinary collaboration, offers the best chance for survival of both mother and fetus.

Maternal resuscitation requires rapid, high-quality CPR adapted to the unique physiological changes of pregnancy, with left uterine displacement to relieve aortocaval compression and early identification of reversible causes. Effective, coordinated teamwork and adherence to established obstetric resuscitation protocols are essential to optimize both maternal and fetal outcomes.

SUGGESTED READING

1. Alimena S, Freret TS, King C, Lassey SC, Economy KE, Easter SR. Simulation to improve trainee knowledge and comfort in managing maternal cardiac arrest. AJOG Glob Rep. 2023;3(2):100182.
2. Del Rios M, Bartos JA, Panchal AR, Atkins DL, Cabañas JG, Cao D, et al. Part 1: executive summary: 2025 American Heart Association Guidelines for Cardiopulmonary Resuscitation and Emergency Cardiovascular Care. Circulation. 2025;152 (Suppl): S284-312.

3. Enomoto N, Yamashita T, Furuta M, Tanaka H, Ng ESW, Matsunaga S, et al. Effect of maternal positioning during cardiopulmonary resuscitation: a systematic review and meta-analyses. BMC Pregnancy Childbirth. 2022;22:159.
4. Jeejeebhoy FM, Zelop CM, Lipman S, Carvalho B, Joglar J, Mhyre JM, et al. Cardiac arrest in pregnancy: a scientific statement from the American Heart Association. Circulation. 2015;132:1747-73.
5. Mushambi MC, Kinsella SM, Popat M, Swales H, Ramaswamy KK, Winton AL, et al. Obstetric Anaesthetists' Association and Difficult Airway Society guidelines for the management of difficult and failed tracheal intubation in obstetrics. Anaesthesia. 2015;70(11):1286-306.
6. Pandya ST, Jain K, Grewal A, Parikh KS, Sharma K, Gupta AK, et al. The Association of Obstetric Anesthesiologists, India–An expert committee consensus statement and recommendations for the management of maternal cardiac arrest. J Obstet Anaesth Crit Care. 2022;12(2):85-93.

19 CHAPTER

Understanding ABG Report

Devang Bharti, Neha Kapoor

INTRODUCTION

Arterial blood gas (ABG) interpretation is a critical clinical skill. It becomes especially relevant when dealing with obstetric emergencies, where rapid physiological deterioration is often encountered. ABG analysis provides crucial information regarding ventilation-oxygenation, and acid-base status, helping clinicians assess severity, plan therapy, and monitor progress. In obstetric practice, any respiratory, circulatory, metabolic, neurological, or major emergency, frequently necessitates rapid ABG assessment **(Table 1)**. To summarize, any obstetric patient with an oxygen saturation of <94% on room air, altered sensorium, suspected lactic acidosis, cardiac disease, or any major emergency requires an ABG analysis.

Pregnancy induces progesterone-driven hyperventilation causing to mild respiratory alkalosis. The partial pressure of carbon dioxide ($PaCO_2$) falls and serum bicarbonate levels (HCO_3^-) decrease to maintain pH. These pregnancy-specific physiological changes must be kept in mind while interpreting ABG in obstetric patients **(Table 2)**.

ENSURING A CORRECT AND RELIABLE ABG REPORT

ABG interpretation is useful only when the sample is collected correctly and analyzed properly. Ensuring the following steps minimize preanalytical errors:

- *Ensuring steady state before sampling*:
  - Changes in oxygen therapy or ventilator setting require at least 30 minutes to reflect in ABG. Longer equilibrium time may be required in chronic respiratory conditions.
- *Following correct sampling technique*:
  - *Preferred site:* Radial artery (after ensuring a positive Allen's test)
  - *Use of appropriate heparinized syringe:* Inadequate heparin may lead to clotting of the sample, while excess heparin causes dilution and falsely lowers $PaCO_2$ values.
  - *Avoiding air bubbles:* Even small air bubbles in the sample may falsely alter PaO_2, decrease $PaCO_2$, and increase pH.

TABLE 1: Indications for performing ABG analysis.

Category	*Clinical situation when indicated*
Assessment of ventilation and oxygenation (suspected or confirmed respiratory compromise)	Acute breathlessness
	Tachypnea
	Hypoxia not responding to oxygen therapy
	Pneumonia/COVID/ARDS
	Suspected pulmonary edema
	Acute exacerbation of asthma
	Assessing need for endotracheal (ET) intubation
	Monitoring response to oxygen therapy/ventilatory adjustments
Hemodynamic instability	Shock (hemorrhagic, septic, cardiogenic)
	Severe APH/PPH
	Suspected lactic acidosis
	Persistent tachycardia with unclear cause
Evaluation of acid-base status	Altered sensorium
	Hyperemesis gravidarum
	Metabolic derangements (e.g., diabetic ketoacidosis, renal failure, sepsis, etc.)
Severe obstetric complications	Pulmonary embolism
	Amniotic fluid embolism
	Severe preeclampsia/eclampsia
	HELLP syndrome
	Abruptio placentae
	Massive obstetric hemorrhage
	Perioperative complications
	Massive blood transfusion
Monitoring in critically ill patients	Mechanical ventilation
	NIV/high-flow oxygen therapy
	Multiorgan dysfunction
	Magnesium toxicity
Anesthesia-related indications	High spinal block
	Delayed recovery following general anesthesia for CS
	Drug-induced hypoventilation
	Intraoperative desaturation

(APH: antepartum hemorrhage; ARDS: acute respiratory distress syndrome; COVID: coronavirus disease; CS: cesarean section; HELLP syndrome: hemolysis, elevated liver enzymes, low platelet syndrome; NIV: noninvasive ventilation; PPH: postpartum hemorrhage)

TABLE 2: Normal ABG values—general and pregnancy.

Parameter	*Normal range*	*Pregnancy range*
pH	7.35–7.45	7.40–7.47
PaO_2 (mm Hg)	80–100	100–105
$PaCO_2$ (mm Hg)	35–45	28–32
HCO_3^- (mEq/L)	22–26	18–21
SaO_2 (%)	>95%	>95%

(ABG: arterial blood gases; HCO_3^-: serum bicarbonate levels; $PaCO_2$: partial pressure of carbon dioxide in arterial blood; PaO_2: partial pressure of oxygen in arterial blood; SaO_2: hemoglobin saturation of arterial blood)

- *Handling the sample appropriately*:
  - Arterial sample should ideally be immediately analyzed, or should be placed on ice if delay is anticipated. Delayed analysis at room temperature rapidly decreases PaO_2 because of blood cell metabolism.
- *Verifying machine input*:
  - Before analyzing the sample, the following parameters should be correctly entered in the machine:
    - FiO_2 (fraction of oxygen in the inspired air)
    - Temperature
    - Hemoglobin concentration
    - Barometric pressure
  - Incorrect values alter the calculated parameters, especially SaO_2, HCO_3^-, etc.

STEP BY STEP ABG SAMPLING TECHNIQUE (RADIAL ARTERY)

- Explain the procedure to the patient and obtain a valid consent.
- Ensure that there are no contraindications, like infection at the puncture site, impaired local circulation, etc.
- Position patient's wrist (preferably non-dominant hand) in supination and slight extension (20–30°), resting it on a rolled towel.
- Perform Allen's test to ensure patency of the ulnar artery for collateral circulation.
- *Prepare the necessary equipment*: Heparinized syringe, alcohol swab, gauze, tape, sharps container, and patient ID label.
- Perform hand hygiene and don appropriate personal protective equipment.
- Cleanse the puncture site with an alcohol or disinfectant swab.
- Palpate the radial artery at the wrist to identify the most pulsatile and superficial site; stabilize the artery between your fingers.

- Warn the patient of the needle prick, then insert the needle at a 30–45° angle (bevel up) just distal to your palpating fingers.
- Advance the needle until arterial blood spontaneously fills the syringe; do not forcefully aspirate with the plunger.
- Withdraw the needle immediately when enough blood is obtained. Apply firm pressure to the site using gauze for at least 3–5 minutes (longer if on anticoagulants).
- Expel air from the syringe, mix the sample gently, and cap the syringe. Label the sample with patient details and send it promptly for analysis.
- Dispose of the needle in the sharps bin, and document the procedure, and any complications.

DETECTING A VENOUS SAMPLE FROM ABG REPORT

At times a venous blood sample may be erroneously sent for ABG analysis. Most of the times this can be detected by corelating the reported values with the clinical condition of the patient.

1. PaO_2 <30–40 mm Hg
2. SaO_2 <75–80%, in a nondesaturating patient
3. $PaCO_2$ >55–60 mm Hg, in a relatively stable patient without underlying chronic obstructive pulmonary disease (COPD).

STEP-WISE APPROACH TO ABG INTERPRETATION

Step 1: Assess Oxygenation

- It helps determine the adequacy of gas exchange and guides immediate clinical decisions, particularly in obstetric emergencies where maternal hypoxemia rapidly compromises fetal oxygen delivery.
- Expected $PaO_2 \approx 5$ times FiO_2 in healthy lungs. A value less than the expected one indicates hypoxemia, and requires oxygen therapy.
- Hypoxemia is classified into mild, moderate and severe, based on the PaO_2 and SaO_2 levels **(Table 3)**. While mild hypoxemia may be managed by administering oxygen through face mask, moderate to severe hypoxemia may require high flow oxygen therapy, noninvasive ventilation (NIV), or ventilatory support through endotracheal (ET) intubation.

TABLE 3: Classification of hypoxemia (at room air: $FiO_2 \approx 0.21$).

Grade	*PaO_2 (mm Hg)*	*SaO_2(%)*
Mild	60–79	90–94
Moderate	40–59	75–89
Severe	<40	<75

(PaO_2: partial pressure of oxygen in arterial blood, SaO_2: hemoglobin saturation of arterial blood)

TABLE 4: Classification of pH abnormalities.

pH Range	*Category*	*Severity classification*
7.35–7.45	Normal	–
<7.35	Acidemia	7.30–7.34: Mild
		7.20–7.29: Moderate
		<7.20: Severe
>7.45	Alkalemia	7.46–7.50: Mild
		7.51–7.54: Moderate
		>7.55: Severe

Step 2: Assess pH

- Assessment of pH establishes the basic acid-base disorder of the patient **(Table 4)**, and guides the subsequent evaluation of the respiratory or metabolic cause.
- Severe acidemia impairs myocardial contractility and predisposes to arrhythmias.
- Severe alkalemia decreases cerebral blood flow, and causes seizures and arrhythmias.
- Fetal acidosis correlates strongly with maternal acidemia, and hence, maternal pH < 7.20 warrants urgent correction.

Step 3: Identify Primary Disorder

- Respiratory disorder: $PaCO_2$ changes in the opposite direction as pH
  - $\uparrow PaCO_2 \rightarrow \downarrow$ pH (respiratory acidosis)
  - $\downarrow PaCO_2 \rightarrow \uparrow$ pH (respiratory alkalosis)
- Metabolic disorder: HCO_3^- changes in the same direction as pH
  - $\downarrow HCO_3^- \rightarrow \downarrow$ pH (metabolic acidosis)
  - $\uparrow HCO_3^- \rightarrow \uparrow$ pH (metabolic alkalosis)
- Mnemonic: ROME—Respiratory Opposite, Metabolic Equal
- In obstetric patients, hyperventilation due to pain, anxiety or early sepsis commonly leads to respiratory alkalosis. Lactic acidosis from hemorrhage or sepsis causes metabolic acidosis. And respiratory depression due to high spinal block, opioid or magnesium toxicity results in respiratory acidosis.

Step 4: Assess the Degree of Compensation

- Acid-base disorders do not exist in isolation for long, as the body starts compensating using the buffer mechanisms.
- Respiratory disorders are compensated using renal buffer mechanisms and metabolic disorders are buffered using pulmonary buffer mechanisms **(Table 5)**.

TABLE 5: Renal and pulmonary compensation.

Disorder	*Event*	*Compensation*
Respiratory acidosis–acute	$PaCO_2$ ↑ 10 mm Hg	1 mEq/L ↑ HCO_3^-
Respiratory acidosis–chronic	$PaCO_2$ ↑ 10 mm Hg	4 mEq/L ↑ HCO_3^-
Respiratory alkalosis–acute	$PaCO_2$ ↓ 10 mm Hg	2 mEq/L ↓ HCO_3^-
Respiratory alkalosis–chronic	$PaCO_2$ ↓ 10 mm Hg	1 mEq/L ↓ HCO_3^-
Metabolic acidosis	1 mEq/L ↓ HCO_3^-	$PaCO_2$ ↓ 1.25 mm Hg
Metabolic alkalosis	1 mEq/L ↑ HCO_3^-	$PaCO_2$ ↑ 0.75 mm Hg

(HCO_3^-: serum bicarbonate level; $PaCO_2$: partial pressure of carbon dioxide in arterial blood)

- Compensation usually does not return pH to normal value, especially in acute disorders. Full compensation suggests chronicity of the disorder or mixed disorders.
- Suspect mixed disorders when:
  - pH is normal but $PaCO_2/HCO_3^-$ are markedly deranged
  - Compensation is inadequate or excessive
  - Clinical picture does not match isolated disturbance

Step 5: Calculate Anion Gap

- Anion gap (AG) helps differentiate types of metabolic acidosis and detect mixed disorders.
- $AG = Na^+ - (Cl^- + HCO_3^-)$
- Normal value: 8–16 mEq/L
- High anion gap metabolic acidosis is commonly seen in lactic acidosis, diabetic ketoacidosis (DKA), renal failure, etc., while normal anion gap metabolic acidosis is encountered in diarrhea, renal tubular acidosis (RTA), etc.

RESPIRATORY ACIDOSIS

Respiratory acidosis results from inadequate alveolar ventilation leading to a primary elevation in $PaCO_2$. Its development indicates the failure of CO_2 excretion to match CO_2 production. A variety of disorders can contribute to this acid-base abnormality **(Fig. 1)**.

It is characterized by:

- pH < 7.35
- $PaCO_2$ > 45 mm Hg
- Compensatory rise in HCO_3^-

The clinical manifestations of acute respiratory acidosis are particularly evident in central nervous system. Since CO_2 readily penetrates the blood brain barrier, and the buffering capacity of the cerebrospinal fluid being not

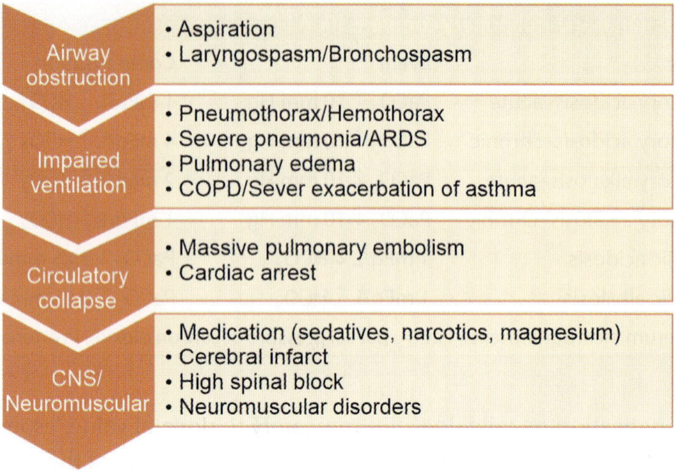

Fig. 1: Causes of respiratory acidosis. (ARDS: acute respiratory distress syndrome; COPD: chronic obstructive pulmonary disease)

as great as blood, a rise in $PaCO_2$ rapidly decreases the pH of the brain. Thus, neurological compromise may be more significant with respiratory acidosis than metabolic acidosis.

Management

- Ensure airway patency
  - Chin lift, jaw thrust
  - Naso/oropharyngeal airway
  - ET intubation
- Improve alveolar ventilation
  - Supplemental oxygen
  - Bag-mask/mechanical ventilation
  - Alteration of ventilator mode/settings
- Treat underlying cause.
  - Bronchodilators for asthma
  - Naloxone for narcotics
  - Calcium gluconate for Magnesium
  - Specific management for other causes

RESPIRATORY ALKALOSIS

Respiratory alkalosis is the result of increased alveolar ventilation, and is frequently seen in pregnancy due to progesterone-mediated hyperventilation. It can also develop pathologically from a variety of causes **(Fig. 2)** including stimulation of brainstem or peripheral chemoreceptors and nociceptive lung receptors.

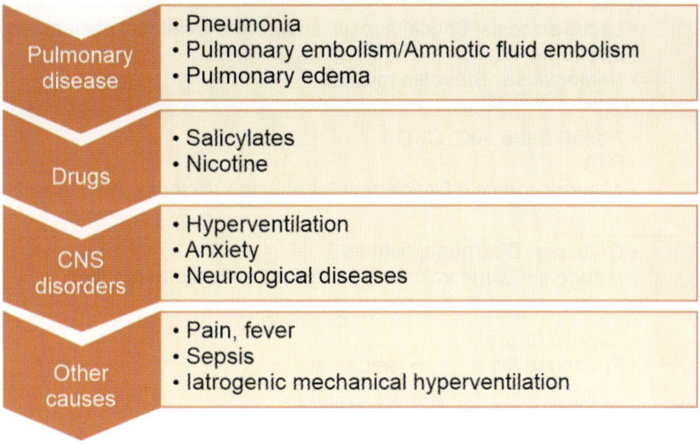

Fig. 2: Causes of respiratory alkalosis.

It is characterized by:

- pH > 7.45
- $PaCO_2$ < 35 mm Hg
- Compensatory fall in HCO_3^-

Management

- Correct hypoxemia
    - Oxygen therapy
    - Airway support, if needed
- Treat underlying cause
- Ventilator adjustments
    - Reduce minute ventilation
- Correct electrolyte disturbances
    - Hypokalemia
    - Hypocalcemia

METABOLIC ACIDOSIS

Metabolic acidosis is one of the most commonly encountered and clinically significant acid-base disturbance in obstetric patients. It can rapidly worsen maternal hemodynamics, and cause fetal acidosis and compromise.

It is characterized by:

- pH <7.35
- HCO_3^- < 22 mEq/L
- Compensatory fall in $PaCO_2$

The physiological hyperventilation during pregnancy allows more efficient respiratory compensation of metabolic acidosis. But this may mask the severity until acidosis becomes profound. The common causes of metabolic acidosis are depicted in **Figure 3**.

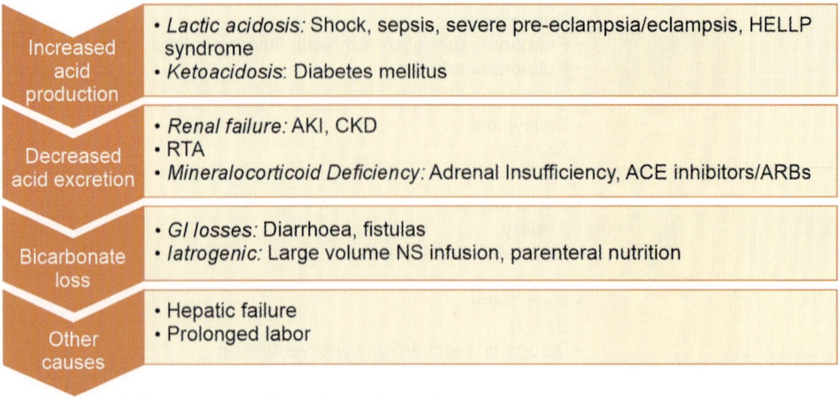

Fig. 3: Causes of metabolic acidosis. (ACE: angiotensin-converting enzyme; AKI: acute kidney injury; ARBs: angiotensin receptor II blockers; CKD: chronic kidney disease; GI: gastrointestinal; HELLP syndrome: hemolysis, elevated liver enzymes, low platelet syndrome; NS: normal saline; RTA: renal tubular acidosis)

Classification

1. *High anion gap metabolic acidosis (HAGMA)*: It is characterized by an AG >16 mEq/L and is commonly encountered in obstetric emergencies, like massive obstetrical hemorrhage, septic shock, amniotic fluid embolism, severe preeclampsia, HELLP syndrome, AKI, DKA, etc.
2. *Normal anion gap metabolic acidosis (NAGMA)*: It is characterized by a normal AG of 8–16 mEq/L and is frequently seen in severe diarrhea, RTA, excessive normal saline (NS) resuscitation, etc.

Management

- Improve tissue perfusion
  - Rapid IV fluid resuscitation
  - Control bleeding
  - Blood transfusion
- Optimize oxygen delivery
  - Supplemental oxygen
  - ET intubation and mechanical ventilation, if required
  - *Correct severe anemia:* Blood transfusion
- Treat underlying pathology
- Judicious use of sodium bicarbonate
  - Indicated only if pH <7.1
  - Ensure adequate ventilation as bicarbonate increases CO_2 load (causes further acidosis)
- 5. Intensive monitoring and complication management

METABOLIC ALKALOSIS

Although less common than metabolic acidosis in obstetric emergencies, metabolic alkalosis frequently occurs in pregnancy-related vomiting and

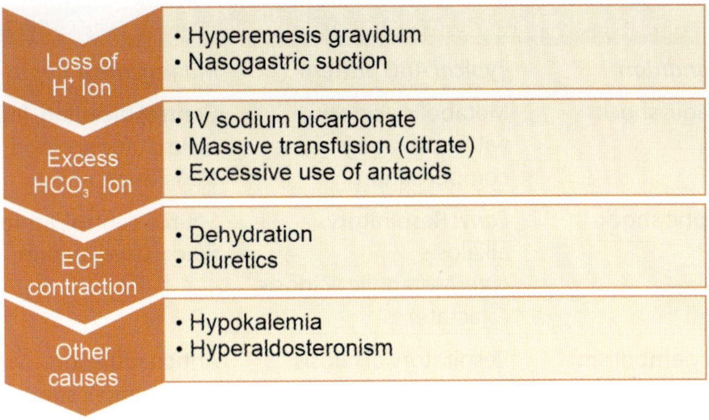

Fig. 4: Causes of metabolic alkalosis. (ECF: extracellular fluid; IV: intravenous)

diuretic use. Persistent alkalosis may impair oxygen delivery and worsen maternal-fetal outcomes.

It is characterized by:

- pH >7.45
- HCO_3^- > 26 mEq/L
- Compensatory rise in $PaCO_2$

The physiological hyperventilation during pregnancy does not cause metabolic alkalosis by itself, but may exaggerate preexisting alkalosis. Its common causes are depicted in **Figure 4**.

Classification

1. Chloride-responsive metabolic alkalosis
   - Urinary Cl^- <15 mEq/L
   - Common in volume depleted states, like vomiting, hyperemesis gravidarum, excess diuretic use.
2. Chloride resistant metabolic alkalosis
   - Urinary Cl^- >20 mEq/L
   - Common in conditions like severe hypokalemia, Cushing's syndrome, primary hyperaldosteronism.

Management

- Restore volume status
  - Correct dehydration
  - Use NS for chloride-responsive metabolic alkalosis
- Correct hypokalemia
- Treat underlying cause

COMMON ABG PATTERNS IN OBSTETRIC EMERGENCIES

ABG patterns and basic management approach for some common obstetric emergencies are listed in **Table 6**.

TABLE 6: Common ABG patterns in obstetric emergencies.

Clinical condition	*Typical ABG pattern*	*Management approach*
Hemorrhagic shock	Metabolic acidosis with respiratory compensation	Control bleeding, fluid resuscitation, blood transfusion
Sepsis/septic shock	*Early:* Respiratory alkalosis *Late:* Metabolic acidosis (↑lactate)	Source control, antibiotics, fluids, oxygenation
Pulmonary embolism	Respiratory alkalosis	Anticoagulation, oxygenation, supportive care
Amniotic fluid embolism	Mixed acidosis	Aggressive resuscitation, oxygenation, vasopressors
High spinal block	Respiratory acidosis	Airway support, ventilatory support, vasopressors
Opioid or magnesium overdose	Respiratory acidosis	Naloxone (for opioids), calcium gluconate (for magnesium), airway support, ventilatory support

(ABG: arterial blood gases)

FINAL INSIGHTS

- ABG interpretation is crucial in obstetric emergencies, where limited physiological reserve can lead to rapid maternal and fetal deterioration.
- A correct ABG interpretation begins with correct sampling and accurate machine handling.
- Never interpret an ABG report without correlating with the accompanying serum electrolyte values.
- Always use a stepwise approach for interpreting ABG: Assess PaO_2 and SaO_2, pH (acidosis or alkalosis), Primary abnormality using $PaCO_2$ and HCO_3^- (respiratory or metabolic), compensation, and anion gap (in case of metabolic acidosis).
- Remember: ROME—Respiratory Opposite, Metabolic Equal
- In obstetrics, common abnormalities include metabolic acidosis from hemorrhage or sepsis, metabolic alkalosis from vomiting or diuretic use, respiratory alkalosis from pulmonary embolism or hypoxia, and respiratory acidosis from high spinal or opioid overdose.
- Management should focus on correcting oxygenation and treating the underlying cause, rather than just normalizing numbers.

SUGGESTED READING

1. Cao Y, Wang M, Yuan Y, Li C, Bai Q, Li M. Arterial blood gas and acid-base balance in patients with pregnancy-induced hypertension syndrome. Exp Ther Med. 2019;17(1):349-53.

2. Chawla S, Jose T, Paul M. Critical Care in Obstetrics: Where are We. J Obstet Gynecol India. 2018;68:155-63.
3. Emmett M. Metabolic alkalosis: a brief pathophysiologic review. Clin J Am Soc Nephrol. 2020;15(12):1848-56.
4. Fenves A, Emmett M. Approach to patients with high anion gap metabolic acidosis: core curriculum 2021. Am J Kidney Dis. 2021;78(4):590-600.
5. Hamilton P, Morgan N, Connolly G, Maxwell A. Understanding acid-base disorders. Ulster Med J. 2017;86(3):161-6.
6. Hamm L, Nakhoul N, Hering-Smith K. Acid-base homeostasis. Clin J Am Soc Nephrol. 2015;10(12):2232-42.
7. Jung B, Martinez M, Claessens Y, Darmon M, Klouche K, Lautrette A, et al. Diagnosis and management of metabolic acidosis: guidelines from a French expert panel. Ann Intensive Care. 2019;9(1):92.
8. Lee G. Clinical applications of blood gas analysis: a comparative review of arterial and venous blood gas monitoring in critical care. Acute Crit Care. 2025;40(2):153-9.
9. Palmer BF, Clegg DJ. Respiratory acidosis and respiratory alkalosis: core curriculum 2023. Am J Kidney Dis. 2023;82(3):347-59.
10. Sarkar M, Niranjan N, Banyal P. Mechanisms of hypoxemia. Lung India. 2017;34(1):47-60.
11. Tinawi M. Pathophysiology, evaluation, and management of metabolic alkalosis. Cureus. 2021;13(1):e12841.

20 CHAPTER

Contents of Eclampsia Tray

Shweta Sardana

INTRODUCTION

Eclampsia is the second most common cause of maternal mortality, and if timely care is provided many complications can be avoided. The eclampsia tray should be available at all the health facilities from primary health care center to an apex tertiary level hospital. A ready Eclampsia tray helps in faster and stress-free management at the time of emergency. The contents of the eclampsia tray can be divided into major subheadings.

DISPOSABLES

1. Sterile gloves—5 pairs **(Fig. 1)**
2. Stethoscope, BP apparatus, knee hammer **(Fig. 2)**
3. Foleys catheter and urine collection bag
4. Urine albumin strips and container **(Fig. 3)**
5. Blood sample collection bottle
6. Spirit swab, IV lines, connectors, IV set, fixation tape
7. Needles and syringes (20 mL, 10 mL, and 5 mL)
8. Distilled water, RL (500 mL), normal saline (100 mL)
9. Tourniquet
10. Suction catheter

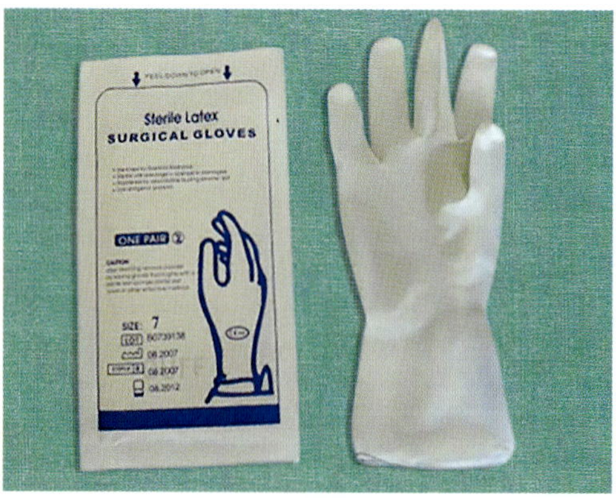

Fig. 1: Sterile gloves.

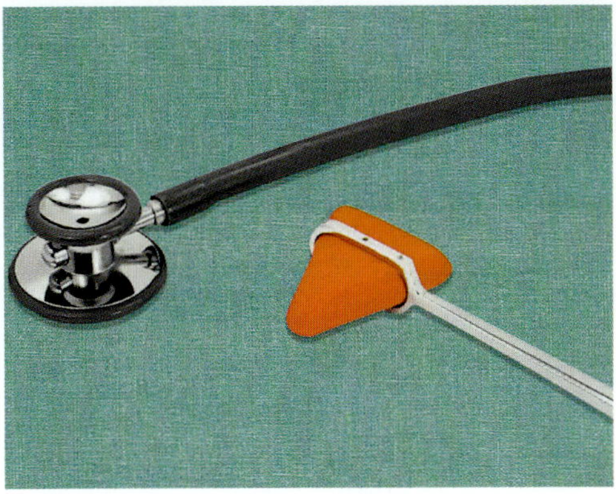

Fig. 2: Stethoscope.

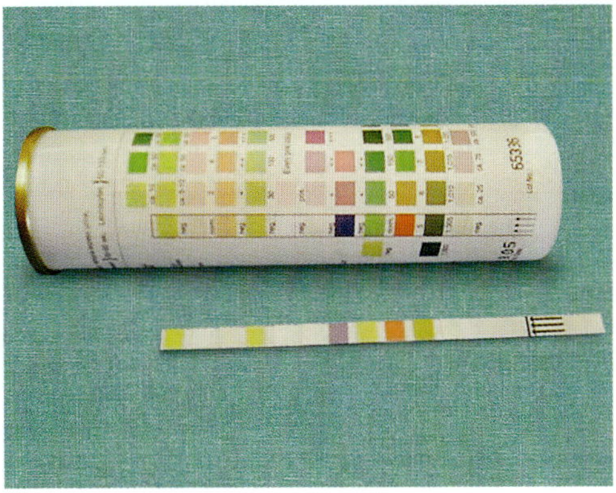

Fig. 3: Urine albumin strips.

11. Guedel airways
12. Face mask and connecting tube for oxygen

MEDICINES

1. Magnesium sulfate ampoules (50%), 2 mL **(Fig. 4)**
2. Calcium gluconate ampoules (10%), 10 mL
3. Injection labetalol 20 mg (4 mL)
4. Injection diazepam **(Fig. 5)**
5. Injection atropine, injection adrenaline, injection Lasix
6. lignocaine jelly

Always check the expiry of the constituents at regular intervals and keep the tray at a readily accessible area. The entire paramedical staff should receive training at regular intervals regarding management of eclampsia patients.

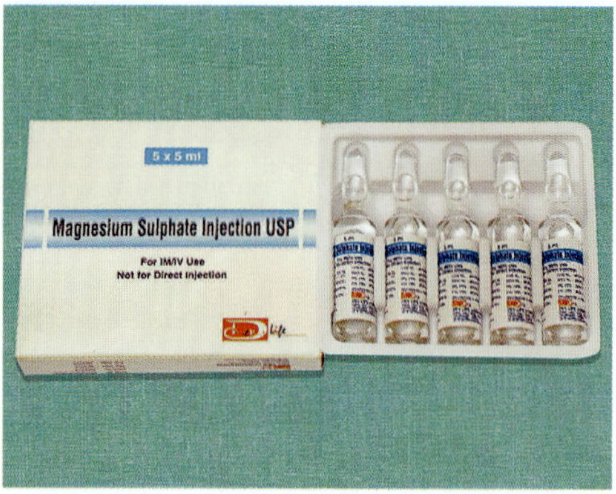

Fig. 4: Magnesium sulfate ampoules.

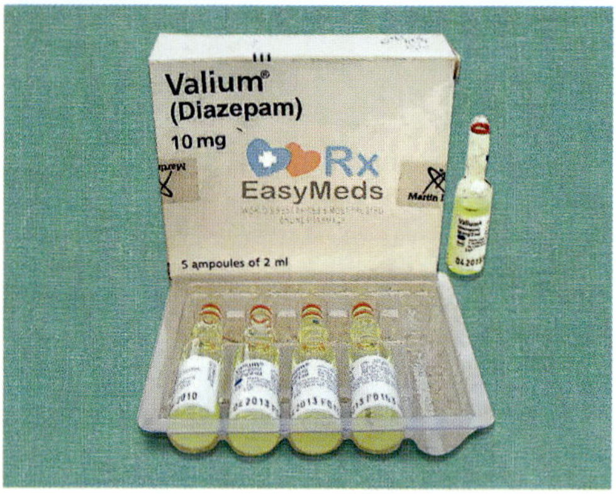

Fig. 5: Injection diazepam.